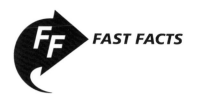

FAST FACTS

C000148043

Managing immune-related Adverse Events in Oncology

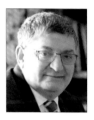

Bernardo L Rapoport MD
Specialist Physician and Medical Oncologist-in-Charge
The Medical Oncology Centre of Rosebank
Saxonwold, Johannesburg
Department of Immunology, Faculty of Health Sciences,
University of Pretoria, Pretoria, South Africa

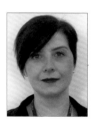

Helen Westman RN MN (Oncology)
Lung Cancer Nurse Coordinator
Cancer and Palliative Care Network
Northern Sydney Cancer Centre
Royal North Shore Hospital
St Leonards, New South Wales
Australia

Declaration of Independence
This book is as balanced and as practical as we can make it.
Ideas for improvement are always welcome: fastfacts@karger.com

KARGER

Fast Facts: Managing immune-related Adverse Events in Oncology
First published 2019
Text © 2019 Bernardo L Rapoport, Helen Westman

© 2019 in this edition S. Karger Publishers Limited

S. Karger Publishers Limited, Elizabeth House, Queen Street,
Abingdon, Oxford OX14 3LN, UK
Tel: +44 (0)1235 523233

Book orders can be placed by telephone (+41 61 306 1440), email
(orders@karger.com) or via the website at: karger.com

Fast Facts is a trademark of S. Karger Publishers Limited.

The rights of Bernardo L Rapoport and Helen Westman to be
identified as the authors of this work have been asserted in
accordance with the Copyright, Designs & Patents Act 1988
Sections 77 and 78.

The publisher and the authors have made every effort to ensure the
accuracy of this book but cannot accept responsibility for any errors
or omissions.

For all drugs, please consult the product labeling approved in your
country for prescribing information.

Registered names, trademarks, etc. used in this book, even when
not marked as such, are not to be considered unprotected by law.

A CIP record for this title is available from the British Library.

ISBN 978-1-912776-39-9

Rapoport BL (Bernardo)
Fast Facts: Managing immune-related Adverse Events in Oncology/
Bernardo L Rapoport, Helen Westman

Medical illustrations by Graeme Chambers.
Typesetting by Thomas Bohm, User Design, Illustration
and Typesetting, UK.
Printed in the UK with Xpedient Print.

List of abbreviations

ACTH: adrenocorticotropic hormone

AKI: acute kidney injury

ALT: alanine transaminase

APC: antigen-presenting cell

AST: aspartate transaminase

CD: cluster of differentiation

CK: creatine kinase

CT: computed tomography

CTCAE: Common Terminology Criteria for Adverse Events

CTLA-4: cytotoxic T lymphocyte-associated antigen 4

DRESS: drug reaction with eosinophilia and systemic symptoms

ECG: electrocardiogram

ED: emergency department

FSH: follicle-stimulating hormone

ICI: immune checkpoint inhibitor

irAE: immune-related adverse event

LH: luteinizing hormone

mAb: monoclonal antibody

MHC: major histocompatibility complex

MRI: magnetic resonance imaging

PD-1: programmed cell death 1 protein

PD-L1: programmed cell death ligand 1

SJS: Stevens–Johnson syndrome

(f)T$_3$: (free) triiodothyronine

(f)T$_4$: (free) thyroxine

TCR: T-cell receptor

TEN: toxic epidermal necrolysis

TFT: thyroid function test

TNF: tumor necrosis factor

TPO: thyroid peroxidase

Treg: regulatory T cell

TSH: thyroid-stimulating hormone

Introduction

The use of immunotherapy for the treatment of both solid and hematologic malignancies is widespread. Immune checkpoint inhibitors in particular have demonstrated considerable promise in the treatment of melanoma, non-small-cell lung cancer and other cancers. Most immune-related adverse events (irAEs) associated with these drugs are mild to moderate, but serious, occasionally life-threatening, adverse events are also reported.

Effective management of irAEs requires early recognition and prompt intervention with steroids, immune suppression and/or immunomodulatory strategies appropriate to the affected organ and severity of toxicity. Educating patients about the potential for, and recognition of, irAEs is also essential.

With immunotherapies becoming more commonplace and healthcare professionals becoming more aware of the benefits of combining immunotherapy strategies, there is a pressing need for guidance on how to recognize and manage the irAEs that may arise.

This resource provides an overview of immuno-oncology and an update on immune checkpoint inhibitors and their associated toxicities, alongside the principles of diagnosing and managing irAEs, important nursing care considerations and a set of convenient management summaries for quick reference. As such, it is essential reading for all members of the cancer care team.

1 Immunotherapy and its side effects: an overview

History

Cancer immunotherapy goes back a century, with the original observations of Paul Ehrlich in 1909. He formulated the hypothesis that host defense may prevent neoplastic cells from developing into tumors: 'In the enormously complicated course of fetal and post-fetal development, aberrant cells become unusually common. Fortunately, in the majority of people, they remain completely latent thanks to the organism's positive mechanisms.'[1]

At the same time, American surgeon William Coley described the association between postoperative infection and improvement of clinical outcomes in patients with cancer.[2] These early observations are a vital foundation for our current understanding and the further development of immune-directed treatments.

Activation and regulation of T-cell responses

Following on from Ehrlich's observations of cancer immuno-surveillance, it is now recognized that the immune system can identify tumor antigens and mount a cytotoxic response via the generation of specific antitumoral cluster of differentiation (CD)8+ T lymphocytes.

Activation of cytotoxic CD8+ T cells encompasses complex interactions that include both T-cell receptor (TCR) signaling and CD28 costimulation (Figure 1.1).[3] 'Signal 1', the interaction between the TCR and foreign antigen presented on major histocompatibility complex (MHC) class I molecules, is not sufficient in itself to enable T-cell activation. 'Signal 2' is provided when the CD28 receptor, which is constitutively expressed on T cells, binds to CD80 (B7-1) and CD86 (B7-2) molecules expressed on antigen-presenting cells (APCs). 'Signal 3' occurs on binding of the MHC class I molecules to accessory CD8 molecules on the T cell (see Figure 1.1).

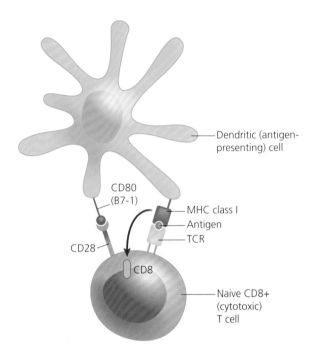

Figure 1.1 Activation of cytotoxic cluster of differentiation (CD)8+ T cells requires three signals: (1) the binding of the T-cell receptor (TCR) to antigen from intracellular pathogens presented on major histocompatibility complex (MHC) class I molecules; (2) the binding of the MHC class I molecules to accessory CD8 molecules on the T cell; and (3) the binding of CD80 (B7-1) on the T cell with CD28 on the antigen-presenting cell. Adapted from Messerschmidt et al. 2016.[4]

Tumor cells are unable to activate T cells directly.[5] Instead, fragments of tumor cells must be phagocytosed by APCs, such as dendritic cells, before antigen processing and presentation by the APCs. T cells then interact with the APCs to receive the signals for T-cell activation, resulting in cytokine production and proliferation as well as the active killing of tumor cells.

Nevertheless, this antitumoral T-cell response ultimately fails for two main reasons: cancer immunoediting and activation of immune checkpoint pathways.[6–8]

Cancer immunoediting

Cancer immunoediting – the process through which the immunogenicity of cancer cells changes – has three phases (the three Es; Table 1.1):

- elimination
- equilibrium
- escape.

The development of central and peripheral immune tolerance, involving the activation of T regulatory cells (Tregs) and other immunosuppressive cells, is crucial for the establishment of the escape mechanism.[7] This process is characterized by crosstalk between the immune cells, cancer cells and the microenvironment. The immune system plays contradictory roles as it protects the host from tumor development but eventually promotes tumor progression.

TABLE 1.1

The three Es of cancer immunoediting

Elimination (of cancer cells)	Activation of the innate and adaptive immune response (NK, CD4+ and CD8+ cells), resulting in the recognition and destruction of tumor cells
Equilibrium (between immune and tumor cells)	Survival of persistent malignant clones/cells. At first, the immune response is sufficient to prevent proliferation, but eventually enough cells are able to avoid the immune response to trigger immunoediting
Escape	Resistant tumor cells evade detection and elimination by the immune system, leading to the: • establishment of low-immunogenic tumors • development of an immunosuppressive microenvironment • appearance of clinically detectable tumors

CD, cluster of differentiation; NK, natural killer [cell].
Source: Dunn et al. 2004.[6]

Activation of immune checkpoint pathways

Tumor cells activate immunosuppressive pathways that inhibit the
initial antitumoral T-cell response via two principal immune
checkpoint molecules expressed on the surface of activated T cells:[9,10]

- the protein receptor cytotoxic T lymphocyte-associated antigen 4
  (CTLA-4)
- the cell surface receptor programmed cell death 1 (PD-1) protein.

CTLA-4. Following the binding of the TCR to an antigen and a
costimulatory signal through the binding of CD28 and CD80, CTLA-4
translocates to the cell surface, where it outcompetes CD28 for
binding to critical costimulatory molecules (CD80, CD86) (Figure 1.2).
This results in inhibitory signaling within the T cell, arresting both
proliferation and activation.

PD-1. The PD-1 receptor on the surface of T cells has emerged as the
primary negative regulator of antitumor T-cell effector function when
it binds to its ligand PD-L1, expressed on the surface of tumor cells
(Figure 1.3). PD-1 has as its ligand programmed cell death ligand 1
(PD-L1 [CD274 or B7-H1]), which is expressed by many somatic cells,
mainly on exposure to proinflammatory cytokines.

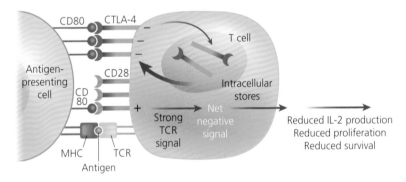

Figure 1.2 Effects of cytotoxic T lymphocyte-associated antigen 4
(CTLA-4) on T-cell function. Binding of cluster of differentiation (CD)80 (B7-1)
on the antigen-presenting cell to CTLA-4 on the T cell in preference to CD28
leads to decreased proliferation and survival of T cells. IL-2, interleukin 2;
MHC, major histocompatibility complex; TCR, T-cell receptor. Adapted from
Buchbinder and Desai 2016.[11]

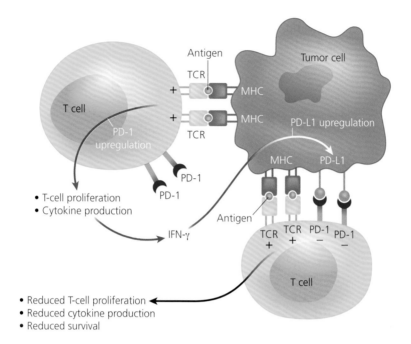

Figure 1.3 Binding of the programmed cell death 1 (PD-1) protein receptor on the surface of T cells to programmed cell death ligand 1 (PD-L1) on the surface of tumor cells leads to the development of T-cell tolerance, with reduced T-cell proliferation, decreased cytokine expression and impaired antigen recognition. IFNγ, interferon γ; MHC, major histocompatibility complex; TCR, T-cell receptor. Adapted from Buchbinder and Desai 2016.[11]

Inflammation-induced PD-L1 expression in the tumor micro-environment leads to PD-1-mediated T-cell exhaustion, with subsequent inhibition of the antitumor cytotoxic T-cell response.[12–14]

Immune checkpoint inhibitors

Blockade of the T-cell checkpoint molecules CTLA-4 and PD-1 and the PD-L1 ligand by immune checkpoint inhibitors (ICIs) has shown remarkably durable clinical responses in a variety of cancers. ICIs essentially take the 'brakes' off the immune system, such that it can once again identify and attack cancer cells. Monoclonal antibodies that bind and inhibit PD-1, PD-L1 and CTLA-4 are available (Figure 1.4; Tables 1.2–1.4 – see end of Chapter).

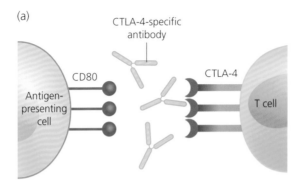

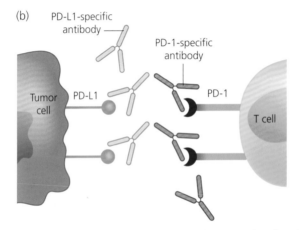

Figure 1.4 Monoclonal antibodies block the ligand/receptor binding that would otherwise lead to inactivation of T cells and tumor escape: (a) cytotoxic T lymphocyte-associated antigen 4 (CTLA-4); and (b) the programmed cell death 1 (PD-1)/programmed cell death ligand 1 (PD-L1).

Immune-related adverse events

Treatment with immune checkpoint inhibitory antibodies is well tolerated by most patients and they are generally less toxic than standard chemotherapy agents. However, when anti-PD-1, anti-PD-L1 and anti-CTLA-4 drugs reactivate the T cells that target cancer cells, they can also cause T cells to attack normal cells (autoimmunity) or can exacerbate immune responses. The resulting side effects are referred to as immune-related adverse events (irAEs),[15] and they include fatigue and dermatologic, gastrointestinal, hepatic, pulmonary and endocrine toxicities. Less common irAEs include diabetes and neurological, ocular, hematologic and cardiac toxicities. Although controversial, reports suggest that irAEs are associated with better outcomes in patients with advanced or recurrent malignancies treated with anti-CTLA-4 and anti-PD-1 therapies.[16]

Immune-related AEs occur relatively early in the course of treatment, with most events happening within weeks to 3 months after initiation of therapy. There are, however, reports of the first documentation of an irAE as long as 1 year after treatment discontinuation.

Once an irAE is documented, a quick work-up is essential, and action should be taken to prevent further intensification.

Skin toxicities can develop after an initial dose of CTLA-4 or PD-1/PD-L1 inhibitor and can be ongoing. The most common rashes are mild, taking the form of maculopapular eruption.[17] Rashes and generalized pruritus are more common with CTLA-4 inhibitor treatment than with anti-PD-1 or anti-PD-L1 (anti-PD-1/PD-L1) therapy.[18]

Rare cases of severe skin reactions such as Stevens–Johnson syndrome and toxic epidermal necrolysis have been described.[19] Vitiligo occurs in a small percentage of patients treated with checkpoint inhibitors and, intriguingly, is associated with long-term survival and clinical benefit.[20]

Gastrointestinal side effects include mucositis, gastritis and colitis. Patients may have diarrhea with blood or mucus. In severe cases, gastrointestinal complications can progress to toxic megacolon and perforation. Other severe complications include peritonitis or *Clostridium difficile* infection.[21]

Pulmonary side effects. Immune-related pneumonitis is a severe complication associated with ICI therapy. It is more common with anti-PD-1 and anti-PD-L1 therapies than with CTLA-4 blockers; however, the incidence of severe pneumonitis is low and it presents later during the treatment phase.[22] New symptoms of dyspnea or cough should alert the clinician to a diagnosis of pneumonitis. This complication could be fatal if not diagnosed promptly.[22]

Endocrine side effects are generally non-specific. They include fatigue, changes in mental state, headaches and dizziness related to hypotension. Hypophysitis and hypothyroidism are the most frequently observed endocrinopathies.[23] Clinicians should screen for thyroid abnormalities at baseline and then at regular intervals. Depending on the type of complaint, other hormone assays may be indicated in some patients.

Other side effects. Ophthalmologic irAEs in the form of mild, moderate or severe episcleritis, uveitis or conjunctivitis have been described.[24] Neurological irAEs include Guillain–Barré syndrome, posterior reversible encephalopathy syndrome, enteric neuropathy, aseptic meningitis, transverse myelitis and mononeuritis multiplex.[25]

Less frequently, hematologic complications may arise in the form of hemolytic–uremic syndrome, red cell aplasia, neutropenia, acquired hemophilia A and thrombocytopenia.[26] Other less frequent side effects include pancreatitis, an asymptomatic rise in amylase and lipase levels, arthritis, renal insufficiency with nephritis, and myocarditis.

Reporting irAEs. Immune-related symptoms are usually low grade and controllable; however, they are often under-reported.[27] Further, irAEs are unpredictable and can be severe. Given the distinctive toxicities associated with immunotherapy, clinicians need to be vigilant.

Combination therapy. Differences in the mechanisms of action of CTLA-4 and PD-1/PD-L1 antibodies have led to investigation of combination regimens in a variety of malignancies, including metastatic renal cell cancer and metastatic malignant melanoma. Around 95% of patients receiving treatment with combination immune checkpoint blockers experience irAEs, with grade 3 or higher toxicities in 50% of these patients. In a Phase III study, severe grade 3 and 4 adverse events were reported in about half of the patients who received combined anti-CTLA-4 and anti-PD-1 therapy, a higher incidence than was reported for either antibody when given separately.[28] As a result, the combined immunotherapy was discontinued in one-third of study participants.

In the future, these agents are likely to be administered concomitantly with targeted therapies, vaccines, chemotherapy or radiation therapy, which will change the incidence and severity of the associated toxicities.

Diagnosing and managing irAEs. Because these side effects can be life-threatening or even fatal, a high level of suspicion should be present while managing patients receiving treatment with checkpoint inhibitors, when atypical or systemic symptoms or signs are detected. Early diagnosis of irAEs and active and aggressive management by the treating clinician is critical to lower morbidity and mortality in patients undergoing treatment with ICIs. However, it is important to note that the clinical recommendations for managing irAEs, as discussed in this book, have been drawn from general clinical consensus and the experience of clinicians with these agents. There are no prospective studies assessing whether one treatment strategy is superior to another.

Management by toxicity grade. The management of each side effect and complication depends on the organ or system involved. As a general rule, ICI treatment should be continued, with close monitoring, for grade 1 toxicities, except for some neurological, hematologic and cardiac toxicities. Therapy with ICIs may be interrupted for most grade 2 toxicities, with treatment restarted when toxicity symptoms revert to grade 1 or full normalization occurs. Grade 2 toxicity can be treated with low-dose corticosteroids.

The management of grade 3 toxicities generally warrants the discontinuation of the ICI(s) and treatment with high-dose corticosteroids (prednisone, 1–2 mg/kg/day, or methylprednisolone, 1–2 mg/kg/day). Corticosteroids should be given for at least 4–6 weeks and then tapered slowly with regular vigilance. Individuals with refractory toxicities may require infliximab (anti-tumor necrosis factor [TNF]) or other immunosuppressive agents.

Additionally, long-term treatment (> 6 weeks) with immunosuppressive drugs increases the chance of opportunistic infections; therefore, pneumocystis prophylaxis should be considered. Thus far, there is no substantial evidence that the clinical outcome of patients receiving treatment with ICIs is affected by the use of immunosuppressive agents for the management of irAEs.

As a general rule, permanent discontinuation of ICIs is recommended for patients with grade 4 toxicities. An exception is the treatment of endocrinopathies that can be controlled by hormone replacement treatment.

TABLE 1.2

Indications for FDA-approved PD-1 checkpoint inhibitors*

Pembrolizumab

Malignant melanoma
- Unresectable or metastatic melanoma
- Adjuvant treatment of melanoma with lymph-node involvement after complete resection

Metastatic non-small-cell lung cancer (NSCLC)
- In combination with pemetrexed and platinum Cx for non-squamous NSCLC with no *EGFR* or *ALK* aberrations – first line
- In combination with carboplatin and paclitaxel or nab-paclitaxel for squamous NSCLC – first line
- NSCLC with high PD-L1 expression (TPS ≥ 50%) and no *EGFR* or *ALK* aberrations – first line
- NSCLC with PD-L1 expression (TPS ≥ 1%) after progression on platinum-containing Cx
- NSCLC with *EGFR* or *ALK* aberrations after progression on approved therapy for these aberrations

Recurrent or metastatic head and neck squamous cell carcinoma
- After progression on platinum-containing Cx

Classic Hodgkin lymphoma (cHL)
- Adults and children with refractory cHL
- Adults and children who have relapsed after ≥ 3 prior lines of therapy

Primary mediastinal large B-cell lymphoma (PMBCL)
- Adults and children with refractory PMBCL
- Adults and children who have relapsed after ≥ 2 prior lines of therapy

CONTINUED

TABLE 1.2 (CONTINUED)

Indications for FDA-approved PD-1 checkpoint inhibitors*

Locally advanced or metastatic urothelial carcinoma
- For tumors with PD-L1 expression (CPS ≥ 10) if ineligible for cisplatin-containing Cx
- If ineligible for any platinum-containing Cx, regardless of PD-L1 status
- During or after platinum-containing Cx or within 12 months of neoadjuvant or adjuvant platinum-containing Cx

Microsatellite instability high (MSI-H) cancer
- Adults and children with unresectable metastatic MSI-H or dMMR solid tumors after progression on prior treatment if there are no alternative treatment options
- Colorectal cancer after progression on treatment with fluoropyrimidine, oxaliplatin and irinotecan

Gastric cancer
- Recurrent locally advanced or metastatic gastric or gastroesophageal junction adenocarcinoma with PD-L1 expression (CPS ≥ 1) after progression on ≥ 2 prior lines of therapy including fluoropyrimidine- and platinum-containing Cx, and, if appropriate, HER2/neu-targeted therapy

Recurrent or metastatic cervical cancer
- With PD-L1 expression (CPS ≥ 1) after progression on or after Cx

Hepatocellular carcinoma
- After treatment with sorafenib

Merkel cell carcinoma
- Adults and children with recurrent locally advanced or metastatic Merkel cell carcinoma

*At the time of publication.
ALK, gene encoding anaplastic lymphoma kinase; CPS, combined positive score; Cx, chemotherapy; dMMR, mismatch repair deficient; *EGFR*, gene encoding epidermal growth factor receptor; FDA, Food and Drug Administration; HER2/neu, human epidermal growth factor receptor 2 (also called erb-b2 receptor tyrosine kinase 2 [ERBB2]; PD-1, programmed cell death 1 protein; PD-L1, programmed cell death ligand 1; TPS, tumor proportion score.

CONTINUED

TABLE 1.2 (CONTINUED)

Indications for FDA-approved PD-1 checkpoint inhibitors*

Nivolumab

Malignant melanoma
- Unresectable or metastatic melanoma as monotherapy or in combination with ipilimumab
- Adjuvant treatment of melanoma with lymph-node involvement or metastases after complete resection

Metastatic non-small-cell lung cancer (NSCLC)
- Progression on or after platinum-containing Cx
- NSCLC with *EGFR* or *ALK* aberrations after progression on approved therapy for these aberrations

Metastatic small-cell lung cancer
- Progression after platinum-containing Cx and ≥ 1 other prior line of therapy

Renal cell carcinoma (RCC)
- Advanced RCC after anti-angiogenic therapy
- In combination with ipilimumab for previously untreated intermediate- or poor-risk RCC

Classic Hodgkin lymphoma (cHL)
- Adults with relapsed or progressed cHL after autologous HSCT and brentuximab vedotin
- Adults with relapsed or progressed cHL after ≥ 3 lines of systemic therapy that includes autologous HSCT

Recurrent or metastatic head and neck squamous cell carcinoma
- Progression on or after platinum-containing Cx

Urothelial carcinoma
- Progression on or after platinum-containing Cx or within 12 months of neoadjuvant or adjuvant treatment with platinum-containing Cx

Hepatocellular carcinoma
- After treatment with sorafenib

CONTINUED

TABLE 1.2 (CONTINUED)

Indications for FDA-approved PD-1 checkpoint inhibitors*

SI-H or dMMR metastatic colorectal cancer
- Adults and children (≥ 12 years) with progression after treatment with fluoropyrimidine, oxaliplatin and irinotecan, as monotherapy or in combination with ipilimumab

Cemiplimab
Locally advanced or metastatic cutaneous SCC
- First-line treatment if ineligible for curative surgery or radiation

*At the time of publication.
ALK, gene encoding anaplastic lymphoma kinase; Cx, chemotherapy; dMMR, mismatch repair deficient; *EGFR*, gene encoding epidermal growth factor receptor; FDA, Food and Drug Administration; HSCT, hematopoietic stem cell transplantation; MSI-H, microsatellite instability high; PD-1, programmed cell death 1 protein; SCC, squamous cell carcinoma.

TABLE 1.3

Indications of FDA-approved PD-L1 checkpoint inhibitors*

Atezolizumab
Locally advanced or metastatic urothelial carcinoma
- With expression of PD-L1 (PD-L1-stained tumor-infiltrating immune cells covering ≥ 5% of tumor area) and ineligible for cisplatin-containing Cx
- Ineligible for any platinum-containing Cx regardless of level of PD-L1 expression
- With progression during or after platinum-containing Cx or within 12 months of neoadjuvant or adjuvant Cx

Metastatic non-small-cell lung cancer (NSCLC)
- With progression during or after platinum-containing Cx
- NSCLC with *EGFR* or *ALK* aberrations after progression on approved therapy for these aberrations

*At the time of publication.
ALK, gene encoding anaplastic lymphoma kinase; Cx, chemotherapy; *EGFR*, gene encoding epidermal growth factor receptor; FDA, Food and Drug Administration; PD-L1, programmed cell death ligand 1.

CONTINUED

TABLE 1.3 (CONTINUED)

Indications of FDA-approved PD-L1 checkpoint inhibitors*

Durvalumab

Locally advanced or metastatic urothelial carcinoma
- Progression during or after platinum-containing Cx or within 12 months of neoadjuvant or adjuvant treatment with platinum-containing Cx

Unresectable stage III non-small-cell lung cancer
- After platinum-containing Cx and radiation therapy if the disease has not progressed

Avelumab

Merkel cell carcinoma
- Adults and children (≥ 12 years)

*At the time of publication.
Cx, chemotherapy; FDA, Food and Drug Administration; PD-L1, programmed cell death ligand 1.

TABLE 1.4

Indications of FDA-approved CTLA-4 checkpoint inhibitor*

Ipilimumab

Malignant melanoma
- Adults and children (≥ 12 years) with unresectable or metastatic melanoma
- Adjuvant treatment of cutaneous melanoma with pathological regional lymph-node involvement > 1 mm after complete resection, including total lymphadenectomy

Renal cell carcinoma (RCC)
- In combination with nivolumab for previously untreated intermediate- or poor-risk advanced RCC

*At the time of publication.
CTLA-4, cytotoxic T lymphocyte-associated antigen 4; FDA, Food and Drug Administration.

Key points – immunotherapy and its side effects: an overview

- Activation of CD8+ cytotoxic T cells requires three signals: engagement of the T-cell receptor (TCR) to antigen presented on major histocompatibility complex (MHC) class I molecules; the binding of CD80 (B7-1) on the T cell with CD28 on the antigen-presenting cell; and the binding of MHC class I molecules to accessory CD8 molecules on the T cell.
- Cancer immunoediting results in resistant tumor cells that evade detection and elimination, leading to the development of clinically detectable cancer.
- Tumor cells activate immunosuppressive pathways that inhibit the initial antitumor T-cell response via immune checkpoint molecules expressed on the surface of activated T cells.
- Immune checkpoint targets for immunotherapy include programmed cell death 1 (PD-1) protein, programmed cell death ligand 1 (PD-L1) and cytotoxic T lymphocyte-associated antigen 4 (CTLA-4).
- Treatment with monoclonal antibodies that bind and inhibit PD-1, PD-L1 and CTLA-4 is well tolerated and generally less toxic than standard chemotherapy.
- Although immune-related adverse events (irAEs) are usually low grade and controllable, they are unpredictable and can be severe, so vigilance is needed.
- Early diagnosis and aggressive management of irAEs is critical to lower morbidity and mortality.

Key references

1. Ribatti D. The concept of immune surveillance against tumors. The first theories. *Oncotarget* 2017;8:7175–80.

2. Hoption Cann SA, van Netten JP, van Netten C. Dr William Coley and tumour regression: a place in history or in the future. *Postgrad Med J* 2003;79:672–80.

3. Beyersdorf N, Kerkau T, Hünig T. CD28 co-stimulation in T-cell homeostasis: a recent perspective. *Immunotargets Ther* 2015;4:111–22.

4. Messerschmidt JL, Predergast GC, Messerschmidt GL. How cancers escape immune destruction and mechanisms of action for the new significantly active immune therapies: helping nonimmunologists decipher recent advances. *Oncologist* 2016;21:233–43.

5. Chen L, Flies DB. Molecular mechanisms of T cell co-stimulation and co-inhibition. *Nat Rev Immunol* 2013;13:227–42.

6. Dunn GP, Old LJ, Schreiber RD. The three Es of cancer immunoediting. *Annu Rev Immunol* 2004;22:329–60.

7. Swann JB, Smyth MJ. Immune surveillance of tumors. *J Clin Invest* 2007;117:1137–46.

8. Corthay A. Does the immune system naturally protect against cancer? *Front Immunol* 2014;5:197.

9. Baitsch L, Fuertes-Marraco SA, Legat A et al. The three main stumbling blocks for anticancer T cells. *Trends Immunol* 2012;33:364–72.

10. Chen DS, Mellman I. Oncology meets immunology: the cancer-immunity cycle. *Immunity* 2013;39:1–10.

11. Buchbinder EI, Desai A. CTLA-4 and PD-1 pathways: similarities, differences, and implications of their inhibition. *Am J Clin Oncol* 2016;39:98–106.

12. Baumeister SH, Freeman GJ, Dranoff G, Sharpe AH. Coinhibitory pathways in immunotherapy for cancer. *Annu Rev Immunol* 2016;34:539–73.

13. Pardoll DM. The blockade of immune checkpoints in cancer immunotherapy. *Nat Rev Cancer* 2012;12:252–64.

14. Ribas A. Adaptive immune resistance: how cancer protects from immune attack. *Cancer Discov* 2015;5:915–19.

15. Baxi S, Yang A, Gennarelli RL et al. Immune-related adverse events for anti-PD-1 and anti-PD-L1 drugs: systematic review and meta-analysis. *BMJ* 2018;360:k793.

16. Ricciuti B, Genova C, De Giglio A et al. Impact of immune-related adverse events on survival in patients with advanced non-small cell lung cancer treated with nivolumab: long-term outcomes from a multi-institutional analysis. *J Cancer Res Clin Oncol* 2019;145:479–85.

17. Sibaud V. Dermatologic reactions to immune checkpoint inhibitors: skin toxicities and immunotherapy. *Am J Clin Dermatol* 2018;19:345–61.

18. Villadolid J, Amin A. Immune checkpoint inhibitors in clinical practice: update on management of immune-related toxicities. *Transl Lung Cancer Res* 2015;4:560–75.

19. Weber JS, Kähler KC, Hauschild A. Management of immune-related adverse events and kinetics of response with ipilimumab. *J Clin Oncol* 2012;30:2691–7.

20. Hua C, Boussemart L, Mateus C et al. Association of vitiligo with tumor response in patients with metastatic melanoma treated with pembrolizumab. *JAMA Dermatol* 2016;152:45–51.

21. Rapoport BL, van Eeden R, Sibaud V et al. Supportive care for patients undergoing immunotherapy. *Support Care Cancer* 2017;25:3017–30.

22. Possick JD. Pulmonary toxicities from checkpoint immunotherapy for malignancy. *Clin Chest Med* 2017;38:223–32.

23. Sznol M, Postow MA, Davies MJ et al. Endocrine-related adverse events associated with immune checkpoint blockade and expert insights on their management. *Cancer Treat Rev* 2017;58:70–6.

24. Antoun J, Titah C, Cochereau I. Ocular and orbital side-effects of checkpoint inhibitors: a review article. *Curr Opin Oncol* 2016;28:288–94.

25. Touat M, Talmasov D, Ricard D, Psimaras D. Neurological toxicities associated with immune-checkpoint inhibitors. *Curr Opin Neurol* 2017;30:659–68.

26. Delanoy N, Michot JM, Comont T et al. Haematological immune-related adverse events induced by anti-PD-1 or anti-PD-L1 immunotherapy: a descriptive observational study. *Lancet Haematol* 2019;6:e48–57.

27. Chen TW, Razak AR, Bedard PL et al. A systematic review of immune-related adverse event reporting in clinical trials of immune checkpoint inhibitors. *Ann Oncol* 2015;26:1824–9.

28. Larkin J, Chiarion-Sileni V, Gonzalez R et al. Combined nivolumab and ipilimumab or monotherapy in untreated melanoma. *N Engl J Med* 2015;373:23–34.

2 Gastrointestinal and hepatic adverse events

Colitis

Mild, self-limiting diarrhea (an increase in stool frequency) is one of the most frequently reported adverse events with immune checkpoint inhibitors (ICIs). The incidence of diarrhea is higher in patients receiving cytotoxic T lymphocyte-associated antigen 4 (CTLA-4) monoclonal antibody (mAb) therapy than in those receiving programmed cell death 1 (PD-1) or programmed cell death ligand 1 (PD-L1) mAb, occurring in 27–54% and 7–18% of patients, respectively.[1-7] Diarrhea of any grade is highest in combination anti-CTLA-4/anti-PD-1 regimens, occurring in up to 44% of patients.[2-9] Similarly, grade 3/4 events are more frequent in patients receiving combination therapy (9%) than in those receiving anti-CTLA-4 or anti-PD-1/anti-PD-L1 monotherapy (3–6% and 0–3%, respectively).[2-9] The common terminology for grading diarrhea toxicities issued by the US National Cancer Institute is shown in Table 2.1.

Diarrhea is a symptom of, but clinically different from, the more serious immune-related gastrointestinal toxicity of colitis. Along with an increase in stool frequency, gastrointestinal toxicity is associated with abdominal pain, watery stools with the presence of mucus or blood, fever, and evidence of inflammation.[10] Diarrhea is the most commonly reported symptom of colitis, occurring – in studies – in 94% of patients who received an anti-CTLA-4 agent[11] and 89% of those using anti-PD-1 therapy.[12] Diarrhea should, therefore, alert clinicians to the possibility of immune-related colitis and prompt appropriate work-up.

Colitis can occur without diarrhea and should not be ruled out in the absence of this symptom. As with diarrhea, the incidence of colitis is more common in combination-treated patients (12–23% of patients, with grade 3/4 severity in 9–17%) and those receiving ipilimumab (8–13% of patients, with grade 3/4 in 3–7%) than in those receiving PD-1 or PD-L1 mAbs, in whom the reported incidence of any grade is less than 4%.[1-6,8-10,13]

24

TABLE 2.1

Grading of severity: diarrhea*

Grade 1

- Increase of < 4 stools/day over baseline
- Mild increase in ostomy output compared with baseline

Grade 2

- Increase of 4–6 stools per day over baseline
- Moderate increase in ostomy output compared with baseline
- Limits instrumental ADL[†]

Grade 3

- Increase of ≥ 7 stools per day over baseline
- Hospitalization indicated
- Severe increase in ostomy output compared with baseline
- Limits self-care ADL[‡]

Grade 4

- Life-threatening consequences
- Urgent intervention indicated

Grade 5

- Death

Bullets within a grade are the equivalent of 'or'.
*A disorder characterized by an increase in frequency and/or loose or watery bowel movements.
[†]Instrumental ADL are the activities and tasks beyond basic self-care that are necessary for living independently; they include activities such as using the telephone, cleaning the house, doing laundry, shopping, going to the bank and managing medications.
[‡]Self-care ADL are bathing, dressing and undressing, self-feeding, using the toilet and taking medications; not bedridden.
ADL, activities of daily living.
Source: Common Terminology Criteria for Adverse Events. National Institutes of Health, National Cancer Institute 2017.[14]

Bowel perforation or colectomy has been reported in 1% of patients with melanoma treated with ipilimumab and a higher proportion of patients with renal cell carcinoma (6.6%). Fatal colitis has been reported in 1%.[1]

The common terminology for grading colitis toxicities issued by the US National Cancer Institute is shown in Table 8.1 (page 74).[14]

Time to onset of immune-related diarrhea and colitis varies, depending on the ICI. The median time to onset for gastrointestinal toxicity has been reported as 1.6 months for combination regimens, with an earlier presentation – 1.4 months – with single-agent ipilimumab.[15] With anti-PD-1 therapy, median time to onset for gastrointestinal toxicity is 7.3 weeks to 3.4 months for nivolumab[3,4,12] and from just under 3 months to 6 months for pembrolizumab.[3,12] However, it is important for clinicians and nurses to be aware that toxicity can develop at any time, as gastrointestinal toxicity has been reported from 0.1 to 37.6 weeks.[9]

Diagnostic evaluation. Immune-related colitis should be considered in any patient using an ICI who presents with diarrhea. Initial work-up should exclude bacterial and viral infective causes.

Physical examination. The evaluation should begin with a thorough head-to-toe assessment to identify the spectrum and severity of symptoms related to enterocolitis, including:
- diarrhea (frequency and consistency)
- presence of blood or mucus in the stools
- abdominal pain
- fever
- vomiting
- mouth ulcers.

Stool culture and testing for *Clostridium difficile*, stool ova and parasites and cytomegalovirus should be undertaken to rule out an infective etiology. Testing for inflammatory markers, such as fecal lactoferrin and fecal calprotectin, may be undertaken where available, though the evidence to support this is varied.[1,16]

Blood tests. Comprehensive blood tests should be performed, including full blood count, electrolytes and renal function, liver function tests, thyroid-stimulating hormone, erythrocyte sedimentation rate and C-reactive protein.

Imaging. For patients presenting with symptoms of grade 2 or higher, abdominal imaging with CT can be a valuable diagnostic tool to identify thickening of the colonic wall. In patients presenting with abdominal pain and fever, abdominal imaging should also be performed to assess for bowel perforation.

To accurately diagnose and evaluate the extent of immune-related colitis, flexible sigmoidoscopy or colonoscopy should be performed. This can be used to assess the presence of ulceration, with biopsies taken to prove histological inflammatory changes; this approach is recommended for patients with persistent diarrhea.[1,3,10,12,15–18]

When to refer. Patients presenting with gastrointestinal toxicity greater than grade 2 should be promptly referred to a specialist gastroenterologist if an infective cause has been excluded. Patients who require investigation with flexible sigmoidoscopy or colonoscopy or management with anti-inflammatory agents, such as the anti-tumor necrosis factor-α agent infliximab, are most appropriately managed by a gastroenterologist who has experience in managing colitis following ICI therapy.

Management of colitis arising from ICI treatment is determined by the severity and grading of symptoms. All patients should be educated about the possible signs and symptoms of colitis and when to alert their healthcare team.

Treatment for grade 2 toxicity or greater is with corticosteroids at a dose of 1 mg/kg/day (prednisone) or methylprednisolone equivalent and can be escalated to 2 mg/kg/day in cases of grade 4 toxicity or grade 2/3 toxicity that does not respond to initial steroid management.

For grade 2 toxicity, ICI treatment should be stopped until symptoms resolve to grade 1. For grade 3, anti-CTLA-4 therapy should be permanently discontinued while restarting anti-PD1 can be considered when symptoms resolve to grade 1.

For grade 4 toxicity, the ICI should be permanently discontinued. Hospitalization should be considered to allow for close monitoring of symptoms as well as management of hydration needs and electrolyte imbalance, as colitis due to ICIs can be fatal. Treatment with infliximab (5 mg/kg) should be started promptly in patients with grade 3 or 4 endoscopy-confirmed colitis if there is no response to high-dose steroids within 3 to 5 days; if needed, a further dose can be administered after 2 weeks (10 mg/kg).[19] Vedolizumab or tacrolimus may also be considered.[20] Management of immune-related colitis is summarized in Table 8.1 (page 74).

Nurses have a vital role in educating patients and carers about the signs and symptoms of immune-related colitis and when to contact their healthcare provider. As nursing staff tend to interact more frequently than doctors with patients and are the initial point of contact for patients being treated with ICIs, they also need to assess, identify and manage gastrointestinal toxicity. Noting a patient's baseline bowel pattern allows early identification of changes, which is important as the Common Terminology Criteria for Adverse Events toxicity grading is based on frequency above baseline.[14] For patients with grade 1 symptoms who are being managed as an outpatient, nurse follow-up is essential for ongoing monitoring of symptoms and rapid escalation of care should symptoms worsen.

Hepatotoxicity

Immune-related hepatitis with an ICI is often asymptomatic and is identified through abnormalities picked up on routine blood tests. Irregular liver function tests, most frequently elevated alanine transaminase and aspartate transaminase (ALT/AST) and, less commonly, bilirubin, occur in up to 30% of patients treated with combination anti-CTLA-4/anti-PD-1 regimens (with grade 3/4 toxicity in ~15%) and 2–10% of patients treated with anti-CTLA-4 (grade 3/4 0–2%) or anti-PD-1/anti-PD-L1 (grade 3/4 1–3%) monotherapy. [2,8,9,13,16,17,21]

Time to onset for hepatotoxicity varies, but symptoms can occur as early as 4 weeks after treatment initiation and as late as 25 weeks. Predominantly, though, hepatotoxicity develops within the first 6–12 weeks of treatment initiation. The common terminology for grading hepatotoxicity is shown in Table 8.2 (page 76).

Diagnostic evaluation

Laboratory work-up. Blood liver function variables (ALT, AST, bilirubin) should be monitored before each ICI infusion. Patients should also be assessed for fatigue and malaise and symptoms of elevated bilirubin, such as jaundice, severe nausea, vomiting and dark-colored urine. Elevated liver enzymes should prompt investigation to exclude other possible etiologies, such as liver metastases, viral hepatitis, thrombosis, drug-induced toxicity or alcohol history.

Imaging. Radiological investigations with liver ultrasound or CT may identify mild hepatomegaly if present but can be helpful to rule out other etiologies.

Biopsy. A liver biopsy can be performed in cases of grade 3 toxicity or when liver function test abnormalities persist.

When to refer. Most cases of immune-related hepatitis respond to corticosteroid management. In cases of grade 3/4 toxicity or those refractory to steroids, referral to a gastroenterologist or hepatologist should be considered.

Management. All patients should be educated about the possible side effects of immune-related hepatitis and should undergo liver function blood tests before each infusion of an ICI.

For grade 1 elevated liver enzymes, the ICI may be continued with close monitoring of liver function – testing once or twice a week. Treatment for grade 2 or greater toxicity is with corticosteroids at a dose of 0.5–1 mg/kg/day (prednisone) or methylprednisolone equivalent. In cases of grade 3/4 toxicity that is not responding to steroid management, consider mycophenolate mofetil. Infliximab is not indicated in the management of hepatitis as its use can result in liver failure.

For grade 2 toxicity, treatment with the ICI should cease until symptoms resolve to grade 1. For more severe toxicities, the ICI should be permanently discontinued. Management of immune-related hepatitis is summarized in Table 8.2 (page 76).

Nurses often review pathology ahead of treatment and undertake pretreatment assessment, so it is essential that nurses know how to interpret liver function blood tests and are familiar with the toxicity grading to ensure appropriate escalation and management.

For patients with grade 1 symptoms who are being managed as an outpatient, nurse follow-up ensures ongoing monitoring of symptoms and prevents delays in management by facilitating rapid escalation of care should symptoms become exacerbated. Nurses also have a key role in educating the patient and carer about signs and symptoms of liver toxicity and when to contact the healthcare team.

Key points – gastrointestinal and hepatic adverse events

- Diarrhea is a symptom of, but is clinically different from, colitis, which may also be associated with abdominal pain, mucus or blood in the stool, and fever.
- Colitis is most frequently reported in patients receiving anti-cytotoxic T lymphocyte-associated antigen 4 (CTLA-4) agents either in combination or as monotherapy.
- Extensive work-up should rule out infective etiologies; colitis should be confirmed by flexible sigmoidoscopy or colonoscopy.
- For colitis, management with infliximab should be initiated promptly if no response to steroids is demonstrated within 3–5 days.
- All patients with grade 2 or higher colitis or grade 3/4 hepatitis should be referred to a gastroenterologist or hepatologist for management.

Key references

1. Gupta A, De Felice KM, Loftus EV Jr, Khanna S. Systematic review: colitis associated with anti-CTLA-4 therapy. *Aliment Pharmacol Ther* 2015;42:406–17.

2. Larkin J, Chiarion-Sileni V, Gonzalez R et al. Combined nivolumab and ipilimumab or monotherapy in untreated melanoma. *N Engl J Med* 2015;373; 1:23–34.

3. Eigentler TK, Hassel JC, Berking C et al. Diagnosis, monitoring and management of immune-related adverse drug reactions of anti-PD-1 antibody therapy. *Cancer Treat Rev* 2016;45:7–18.

4. Weber JS, Hodi FS, Wolchok JD et al. Safety profile of nivolumab monotherapy: a pooled analysis of patients with advanced melanoma. *J Clin Oncol* 2017;35:785–91.

5. Rittmeyer A, Barlesi F, Waterkamp D et al. Atezolizumab versus docetaxel in patients with previously treated non-small-cell lung cancer (OAK): a phase 3, open label, multicentre randomised controlled trial. *Lancet* 2017;389: 255–65.

6. Rosenberg JE, Hoffman-Censits J, Powles T et al. Atezolizumab in patients with locally advanced and metastatic urothelial carcinoma who have progressed following treatment with platinum based chemotherapy: a single arm, multicentre, phase 2 trial. *Lancet* 2016;387:1909–20.

7. Antonia SJ, Villegas A, Daniel D et al. Durvalumab after chemoradiotherapy in stage III non-small-cell lung cancer. *N Engl J Med* 2017;377:1919–29.

8. Sznol M, Ferrucci PF, Hogg D et al. Pooled analysis safety profile of nivolumab and ipilimumab combination therapy in patients with advanced melanoma. *J Clin Oncol* 2017;35:3815–22.

9. Nagai H, Muto M. Optimal management of immune-related adverse events resulting from treatment with immune checkpoint inhibitors: a review and update. *Int J Clin Oncol* 2018;23:410–20.

10. Puzanov I, Diab A, Abdallah K et al. Managing toxicities associated with immune checkpoint inhibitors: consensus recommendations from the Society for Immunotherapy of Cancer (SITC) Toxicity Management Working Group. *J Immunother Cancer* 2017;5:95.

11. Marthey L, Mateus C, Mussini C et al. Cancer immunotherapy with anti CTLA-4 monoclonal antibodies induces an inflammatory bowel disease. *J Crohns Colitis* 2016;10: 395–401.

12. Gonzalez RS, Salaria SN, Bohannon CD et al. PD-1 inhibitor gastroenterocolitis: case series and appraisal of 'immunomodulatory gastroenterocolitis'. *Histopathology* 2017;70:558–67.

13. Postow M, Chesney J, Pavlick A et al. Nivolumab and ipilimumab versus ipilimumab in untreated melanoma. *N Engl J Med* 2015;372:2006–17.

14. National Institutes of Health, National Cancer Institute. Common Terminology Criteria for Adverse Events (CTCAE) v.5, November 2017. https://ctep.cancer.gov/protocol development/electronic_applications/ docs/CTCAE_v5_Quick_Reference_ 8.5x11.pdf, last accessed 2 April 2019.

15. Dadu R, Zobniw C, Diab A. Managing adverse events with immune checkpoint agents. *Cancer J* 2016;22:121–9.

16. Haanen JBAG, Carbonnel F, Robert C et al. Management of toxicities from immunotherapy: ESMO Clinical Practice Guidelines for diagnosis, treatment and follow-up. *Ann Oncol* 2017;28(suppl 4):iv119–42.

17. Brahmer JR, Lacchetti C, Schneider BJ et al. Management of immune-related adverse events in patients treated with immune checkpoint inhibitor therapy: American Society of Clinical Oncology Clinical Practice Guideline. *J Clin Oncol* 2018;36:1714–68.

18. Winer A, Bodor JN, Borghaei H. Identifying and managing the adverse effects of immune checkpoint blockade. *J Thorac Dis* 2018;10(suppl 3):S480–9.

19. Johnston RL, Lutzky J, Chodhry A, Barkin JS. Cytotoxic T-lymphocyte-associated antigen 4 antibody-induced colitis and its management with infliximab. *Dig Dis Sci* 2009;54:2538–40.

20. Som A, Mandaliya R, Alsaadi D et al. Immune checkpoint inhibitor-induced colitis: a comprehensive review. *World J Clin Cases* 2019;7:405–18.

21. Weber JS, Kähler KC, Hauschild A. Management of immune-related adverse events and kinetics of response with ipilimumab. *J Clin Oncol* 2012;30:2691–7.

3 Dermatologic adverse events

Dermatologic toxicities are the second most commonly reported immune-related adverse events (irAEs) from immune checkpoint inhibitors (ICIs) after fatigue, and have the earliest reported onset, typically occurring within the first month of treatment. The incidence of cutaneous irAEs of any grade is highest in patients receiving monoclonal antibodies (mAbs) against combination cytotoxic T lymphocyte-associated antigen 4 (CTLA-4)/programmed cell death 1 (PD-1) and is reported in 59–64% of patients.[1,2] With anti-CTLA-4 and anti-PD-1/PD-L1 monotherapy, the incidence is 44–54%[2,3] and 29–42%, respectively.[2-5]

Skin irAEs are most frequently low grade; serious irAEs requiring discontinuation of therapy are rare. Grade 3/4 toxicities are reported in ~7% of patients receiving combination anti-CTLA-4/anti-PD-1 mAbs, less than 5% of patients treated with anti-CTLA-4 monotherapy[2,3] and less than 1% of patients receiving anti-PD-1/PD-L1 monotherapy.[4,6]

The most common skin toxicities are rash, pruritus and vitiligo. Rarer skin irAEs, including psoriasis, photosensitivity reaction, Stevens–Johnson syndrome (SJS), toxic epidermal necrolysis (TEN) and Sweet's syndrome, have also been reported.[7-9]

Rash

A non-defined rash is reported in ~40% of patients receiving combination ipilimumab/nivolumab therapy, ~24% of patients receiving ipilimumab monotherapy and ~15% of patients treated with anti-PD-1/PD-L1 monotherapy. A grade 3/4 rash is reported in less than 5% of patients using combination therapy and less than 3% of those using ipilimumab or anti-PD-1 monotherapy.[1,4,10,11] The rash, often described as reticular and erythematous, occurs predominantly on the trunk and extremities; it may be asymptomatic or associated with pruritus.[12,13]

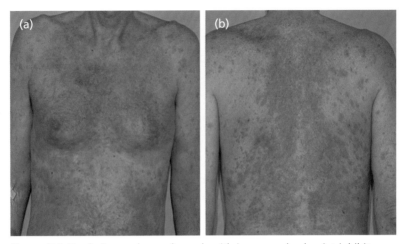

Figure 3.1 Grade 3 maculopapular rash with immune checkpoint inhibitor therapy. Reprinted, by permission from Springer, from Sibaud 2018.[14]

A more specific maculopapular rash (Figure 3.1) has been reported in ~15% of patients receiving combination ICIs, ~8% receiving anti-CTLA-4 monotherapy and ~5% using anti-PD-1/PD-L1 monotherapy, with grade 3/4 events reported in less than 3% of cases.[1,10] The National Cancer Institute's Common Terminology Criteria for Adverse Events (CTCAE) for this type of rash are given in Table 8.3 (page 78).

Pruritus
The incidence of pruritus of any grade is similar to that of a rash, occurring in ~33% of patients on combination therapy, 25–35% of those on ipilimumab monotherapy and 13–20% of those using anti-PD-1/PD-L1 monotherapy.[10,11] Pruritus, which is mostly low grade (< 2% reported grade 3/4), can be localized or more diffuse, with associated skin changes such as lichenification, excoriation and ooze.[12,13] The common terminology for grading pruritus is given in Table 8.4 (page 79).

Vitiligo
Vitiligo (Figure 3.2) occurs predominantly in patients treated for melanoma and it seems to have a positive association with long-term survival, with its presence indicating clinical response to anti-PD-1

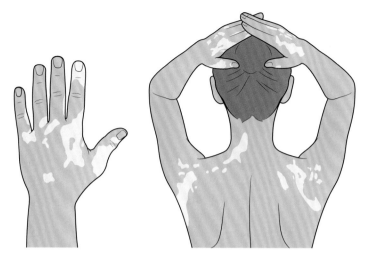

Figure 3.2 Patchy lesions of vitiligo; the grade of severity depends on the body surface area affected.

immunotherapy.[15] Vitiligo has been reported in 8–10% of patients receiving combination ICIs or anti-PD-1 monotherapy; it is less common with single-agent ipilimumab (4%).[10] Vitiligo lesions can persist after treatment discontinuation. The common terminology for grading hypopigmentation, including vitiligo, is given in Table 3.1.

TABLE 3.1

Grading of severity: hypopigmentation*

Grade 1

- Hypopigmentation or depigmentation covering < 10% BSA
- No psychosocial impact

Grade 2

- Hypopigmentation or depigmentation covering > 10% BSA
- Associated psychosocial impact

Bullets within a grade are the equivalent of 'or'.
*A disorder characterized by loss of skin pigment (e.g. vitiligo).
BSA, body surface area.
Source: Common Terminology Criteria for Adverse Events. National Institutes of Health, National Cancer Institute 2017.[16]

Bullous pemphigoid

Immune-related bullous pemphigoid has been reported with the use of PD-1/PD-L1 mAbs and can occur following months of treatment.[14] Bullous pemphigoid blisters are commonly preceded by a maculopapular rash and pruritus. A scheme for grading bullous dermatoses, including bullous pemphigoid and other autoimmune bullous dermatoses, is shown in Table 8.5 (page 80).[16]

Rarer skin immune-related adverse events

Cases of rarer skin irAEs have been reported with the use of both CTLA-4 and PD-1 ICIs. While the incidence needs to be determined, cases of extensive exfoliative dermatitis, SJS and TEN have been described. A maculopapular rash may be the initial presenting symptoms of a more severe dermatologic irAE.[14] The development of psoriasis or exacerbation of pre-existing psoriasis has been reported with both CTLA-4 and PD-1 ICIs and several cases of Sweet's syndrome have been reported in patients treated with ipilimumab.[14] Cases of drug reaction with eosinophilia and systemic symptoms (DRESS) have also been reported. Table 3.2 provides a full spectrum of skin toxicities from ICIs that have been described within the literature.

Diagnostic evaluation

While dermatologic toxicities are one of the most commonly reported irAEs from ICIs, other possible etiologies should be excluded. Differential diagnoses include infection, reaction to another drug, exacerbation of a pre-existing skin disorder and an unrelated skin condition.

Physical examination. A head-to-toe assessment should be performed, including inspection of the patient's mucous membranes. In order to accurately grade the toxicity, a full body examination using an assessment tool should be performed to determine the percentage of body surface area affected (Figure 3.3). Photographic documentation is also helpful for tracking the progress of cutaneous AEs.

Laboratory work-up. Blood tests should be undertaken, including a full blood count, liver and kidney function tests and electrolytes. Further tests, such as a screening antinuclear antibody test, can be performed if an autoimmune condition is suspected.[17]

TABLE 3.2

Spectrum of reported dermatologic toxicities from ICIs

- Eruptive keratoacanthoma
- Actinic keratosis and squamous cell carcinoma
- Erythema-nodosum-like panniculitis
- Radiosensitization
- Grover's disease
- Neutrophilic dermatoses (Sweet's syndrome, pyoderma gangrenosum)
- Dermatomyositis
- Sjögren's syndrome
- Necrotizing vasculitis
- Acneiform eruption
- Papulopustular rosacea
- Annular granuloma
- Peritumoral inflammatory cellulitis
- Toxic epidermal necrolysis, Stevens–Johnson syndrome
- Drug reaction with eosinophilia and systemic symptoms (DRESS)
- Erythema multiforme
- Photosensitivity
- Urticaria
- Alopecia, hair repigmentation
- Sclerodermoid reaction
- Nail changes

ICI, immune checkpoint inhibitor.
Source: Sibaud 2018.[14]

Biopsy. For patients undergoing work-up for suspected bullous dermatoses or more severe cutaneous reaction such as SJS/TEN, a skin biopsy is needed. Skin biopsies should also be taken for patients with a persistent, recurrent or atypical rash.[14]

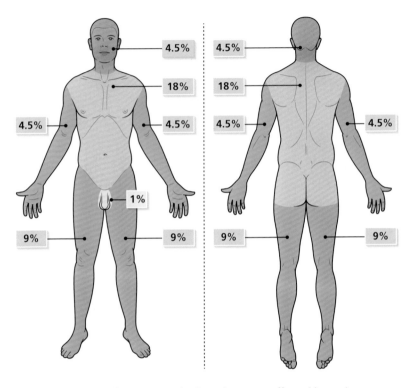

Figure 3.3 A guide for assessing body surface area affected by an immune-related dermatologic adverse event.

For severe cutaneous reactions such as SJS, patients should:
- have blood cultures if febrile
- have regular vital signs taken
- be monitored for additional symptoms such as fevers, photophobia, odynophagia (pain on swallowing), dysuria, pain involving the genitals, abdominal pain or pain associated with bowel movements.[17]

When to refer
Patients who have a suspected dermatologic emergency such as SJS/ TEN, Sweet's Syndrome or DRESS should be admitted to hospital, with urgent referral to a dermatologist. Patients may also require management by a specialized burns unit. In cases of other cutaneous toxicities that are grade 3/4, same-day dermatologist consultation is

recommended. In cases of persistent or worsening grade 2 toxicity, referral to a specialist dermatologist should be considered.

Management

A number of strategies can be put in place to help reduce the risk of developing a skin toxicity or assist in minimizing the exacerbation of cutaneous irAEs, including:[18]

- avoiding sun exposure
- using non-irritant moisturizers
- using mild skin washes
- avoiding scrubbing the skin
- avoiding wearing tight-fitting clothing.

Management depends on toxicity and grade, with topical corticosteroids used for grade 1–2 irAEs, escalating to systemic corticosteroids for grade 3 toxicities. In cases of rash or pruritus, treatment with ICIs may continue with grade 1–2 toxicities but should be stopped in cases of grade 3 toxicity and restarted in consultation with a dermatologist. Where severe and potentially life-threatening cutaneous irAEs are suspected (SJS/TENS, DRESS, Sweet's syndrome), ICI treatment should be stopped immediately.[5,17]

Guidance for managing cutaneous AEs is summarized in Tables 8.3–8.5 (pages 78–81). A steroid-refractory patient should be managed by an experienced dermatologist.

Nursing considerations

Nurses are vital for providing education to patients and carers about the signs and symptoms of cutaneous toxicities as well as skin care and self-management strategies.

As nursing staff are well placed to undertake regular assessment of the patient's skin before each treatment, they have an important role in assessing, identifying and managing dermatologic irAEs. For patients with low-grade symptoms who are being managed as an outpatient and those who are tapering steroids, follow-up by a member of the nursing team enables the ongoing monitoring of symptoms and ensures rapid escalation of care on exacerbation of symptoms. Skin irAEs often impact a patient's quality of life, which may affect treatment adherence – nurses are able to help in these circumstances by providing practical advice using management algorithms.[19]

Key points – dermatologic adverse events

- Dermatologic toxicities are one of the most commonly reported adverse events associated with the use of immune checkpoint inhibitors (ICIs).
- Onset usually occurs within the first 4–8 weeks of initiating therapy.
- Rash and pruritus are the most frequently reported skin toxicities; importantly, they may also be the presenting symptoms of more severe dermatologic conditions.
- All patients with toxicity greater than grade 2 should be referred to a specialist dermatologist; specialist advice should guide decisions on when to restart ICI therapy.
- Nurses have a vital role in assessing the patient and providing education and advice to manage symptoms and maintain quality of life.

Key references

1. Sznol M, Ferrucci PF, Hogg D et al. Pooled analysis safety profile of nivolumab and ipilimumab combination therapy in patients with advanced melanoma. *J Clin Oncol* 2017;35:3815–22.

2. Larkin J, Chiarion-Sileni V, Gonzalez R et al. Combined nivolumab and ipilimumab or monotherapy in untreated melanoma. *N Engl J Med* 2015;373:23–34.

3. Bertrand A, Kostine M, Barnetche T et al. Immune related adverse events associated with anti-CTLA-4 antibodies: systematic review and meta-analysis. *BMC Med* 2015;13:211.

4. Weber JS, Hodi FS, Wolchok JD et al. Safety profile of nivolumab monotherapy: a pooled analysis of patients with advanced melanoma. *J Clin Oncol* 2017;35:785–91.

5. Puzanov I, Diab A, Abdallah K et al. Managing toxicities associated with immune checkpoint inhibitors: consensus recommendations from the Society for Immunotherapy of Cancer (SITC) Toxicity Management Working Group. *J Immunother Cancer* 2017;5:95.

6. Bellmunt J, de Wit R, Vaughn DJ et al. Pembrolizumab as second-line therapy for advanced urothelial carcinoma. *N Engl J Med* 2017;376:1015–26.

7. Nagai H, Muto M. Optimal management of immune-related adverse events resulting from treatment with immune checkpoint inhibitors: a review and update. *Int J Clin Oncol* 2018;23:410–20.

8. Eigentler TK, Hassel JC, Berking C et al. Diagnosis, monitoring and management of immune-related adverse drug reactions of anti-PD-1 antibody therapy. *Cancer Treat Rev* 2016;45:7–18.

9. Pintova S, Sidhu H, Friedlander PA, Holcombe RF. Sweet's syndrome in a patient with metastatic melanoma after ipilimumab therapy. *Melanoma Res* 2013;23:498–501.

10. Postow M, Chesney J, Pavlick A et al. Nivolumab and ipilimumab versus ipilimumab in untreated melanoma. *N Engl J Med* 2015;372:2006–17.

11. Haanen JBAG, Carbonnel F, Robert C et al. Management of toxicities from immunotherapy: ESMO Clinical Practice Guidelines for diagnosis, treatment and follow-up. *Ann Oncol* 2017;28(suppl 4):iv119–42.

12. Habre M, Habre S, Kourie HR. Dermatologic adverse events of checkpoint inhibitors: what an oncologist should know. *Immunotherapy* 2016;8:1437–46.

13. Lacouture ME, Wolchok JD, Yosipovitch G et al. Ipilimumab in patients with cancer and the management of dermatologic adverse events. *J Am Acad Dermatol* 2014;71:161–9.

14. Sibaud V. Dermatologic reactions to immune checkpoint inhibitors: skin toxicities and immunotherapy. *Am J Clin Dermatol* 2018;19:345–61.

15. Hua C, Boussemart L, Mateus C et al. Association of vitiligo with tumor response in patients with metastatic melanoma treated with pembrolizumab. *JAMA Dermatol* 2016;152:45–51.

16. National Institutes of Health, National Cancer Institute. Common Terminology Criteria for Adverse Events (CTCAE) v.5, November 2017. https://ctep.cancer.gov/protocoldevelopment/electronic_applications/docs/CTCAE_v5_Quick_Reference_8.5x11.pdf, last accessed 2 April 2019.

17. Brahmer JR, Lacchetti C, Schneider BJ et al. Management of immune-related adverse events in patients treated with immune checkpoint inhibitor therapy: American Society of Clinical Oncology Clinical Practice Guideline. *J Clin Oncol* 2018;36:1714–68.

18. Dadu R, Zobniw C, Diab A. Managing adverse events with immune checkpoint agents. *Cancer J* 2016;22:121–9.

19. Thebeau M, Rubin K, Hofmann M et al. Management of skin adverse events associated with immune checkpoint inhibitors in patients with melanoma: a nursing perspective. *J Am Assoc Nurse Pract* 2017;29:294–303.

4   Endocrine-related adverse events

Immune-related adverse events (irAEs) that result in alterations to endocrine function are frequently reported, with the endocrine glands most commonly affected being the thyroid, pituitary and adrenal glands. The onset of endocrine toxicity typically occurs within the first 12 weeks of starting therapy with an immune checkpoint inhibitor (ICI). Unlike other irAEs, endocrine-associated adverse events persist despite completion or discontinuation of treatment; they require long-term management with hormone therapy as the affected gland rarely recovers function.[1-4]

Epidemiology

Incidence can be difficult to determine accurately because of the non-specific nature of symptoms, such as fatigue, headaches and nausea. These are symptoms that commonly result from malignancy, sites of metastatic disease and other anticancer and supportive therapies, and their non-specific nature results in the under-reporting or under-detection of endocrine toxicities.[5,6] Grading endocrine toxicity with the Common Terminology Criteria of Adverse Events (CTCAE)[7] may prove insufficient as the Criteria rely on symptoms to determine severity rather than the results of biochemically diagnostic tests.[4,8,9] Incidence may also be difficult to determine accurately as baseline screening for endocrine abnormalities is not routinely undertaken before starting an ICI.

As with other irAEs, the incidence of endocrine toxicity of any grade is highest in those patients treated with combination ICI therapy (~30%).[3] In patients receiving treatment with monotherapy anti-cytotoxic T lymphocyte-associated antigen 4 (CTLA-4) or anti-programmed cell death 1 (PD-1) agents, the incidence of endocrine irAEs is less frequent, reported as ~15% and ~10%, respectively.[1,2,10-12]

Reports of grade 3/4 endocrine toxicities are rare, even with combination therapy (< 5%); however, grade 5 endocrine events have been reported, with one pooled analysis of experience with combination ICI therapy reporting a death from panhypopituitarism with severe adrenal deficiency and adrenal crisis.[3] Grading definitions for endocrine AEs are shown in Tables 8.6–8.10 (pages 82–9).

Diagnostic evaluation

Diagnostic evaluation of endocrine toxicity can be complicated by the lack of baseline screening for endocrine disorders as well as the non-specific and vague nature of symptoms that are also common in patients with advanced cancer. Administration of corticosteroids to treat other irAEs or symptoms of cancer and treatments can interfere with biochemical endocrine tests.[5]

Physical examination. Thorough ongoing assessment for clinical signs and symptoms related to endocrine irAEs should be undertaken in the context of the patient's history and disease state.

Biochemical tests should be performed ahead of treatment, with all patients having thyroid function tests (TFTs) – thyroid-stimulating hormone (TSH), free triiodothyronine (fT$_3$) and free thyroxine (fT$_4$) – and blood glucose monitoring, as well as routine electrolyte evaluation, before each infusion. Adrenal function tests – adrenocorticotropic hormone (ACTH) and cortisol (early morning) – should be performed at baseline and at ongoing regular intervals; cortisol levels should not be routinely checked in patients on corticosteroids as the results cannot be accurately interpreted. Determining whether the hormonal deficiency is primary (damage to the thyroid gland) or secondary (dysfunction of the pituitary gland) is important because of the associated treatment implications; assessment of both the thyroid and pituitary hormone levels should be undertaken.

Primary thyroid dysfunction

Abnormalities of thyroid gland function, most commonly evidence of hypothyroidism, are the most frequently reported endocrine irAEs; they are very rarely severe. Thyroid dysfunction can occur at any time during treatment with ICIs.

Hypothyroidism of any grade is most frequently seen in patients treated with combination ICI therapy (~15%), with grade 3/4 events reported in less than 0.2% of patients.[3,10] The incidence of hypothyroidism is higher in patients treated with PD-1 or programmed death ligand 1 (PD-L1) monoclonal antibody (mAb) monotherapy than in those using single-agent ipilimumab (anti-CTLA-4), being reported in 4–10% and 4–7%, respectively, with no grade 3/4 events reported.[10,11,13]

Hyperthyroidism (thyrotoxicosis) of any grade is less common and has been reported in ~10% of combination-treated patients and 2–7% and 1–2% of patients receiving monotherapy with either anti-PD-1/ PD-L1 or ipilimumab, respectively. Grade 3/4 events are reported in less than 1% of patients.[3,11] In one study, subclinical hyperthyroidism was reported in 22% of patients treated with combination ICI therapy, 16% of ipilimumab-treated patients and 13% of patients receiving PD-1 mAb therapy; however, the overall incidence of subclinical hypo/ hyperthyroidism is likely to be difficult to determine accurately.[14] The most common cause of thyrotoxicosis is thyroiditis, which is self-limiting and leads to permanent hypothyroidism.

Diagnostic evaluation of thyroid dysfunction should include both a thorough clinical assessment of signs and symptoms associated with hypo/hyperthyroidism and a biochemical assessment, with TSH, fT_3 and fT_4 levels being checked before each ICI infusion.

Hypothyroidism. Symptoms of hypothyroidism include fatigue, weight gain, hair loss, constipation and intolerance to cold. These symptoms should be recorded, with particular attention paid to the overall trend of symptoms (such as incremental weight gain) and consideration given to other potential etiologies.

Biochemically, high TSH and low T_4 levels indicate primary hypothyroidism; these findings should be followed by additional testing for thyroid antibodies, such as antithyroid peroxidase (TPO).

Hyperthyroidism (thyrotoxicosis) symptoms include weight loss, palpitations, heat intolerance, anxiety and diarrhea. It can be confirmed with laboratory testing, with patients having high levels of fT_4 or fT_3 with low or normal TSH. Further tests, including TSH receptor antibody or thyroid-stimulating immunoglobulin and TPO, should then be considered if clinical features of Graves' disease are present. In the case of hyperthyroidism, thyroid function should be monitored closely because of the likelihood of transitioning to hypothyroidism.[5,9,14-16]

Hypophysitis

Hypophysitis (inflammation of the pituitary gland) is most commonly seen with ipilimumab-containing regimens (10–13% with monotherapy, < 11% with combination regimens); it is rare with PD-1/PD-L1 checkpoint inhibition (< 1%).[2,10,13,15] With onset typically within the first 9 weeks of treatment, hypophysitis can lead to a range of disorders resulting from low levels of all or some of the pituitary gland hormones. These include ACTH, TSH and luteinizing hormone (LH).

Diagnostic evaluation of hypophysitis should include a clinical assessment of symptoms, biochemical evaluation of anterior pituitary hormones and diagnostic imaging of the brain.

Symptoms. The most common symptoms are headache (85%) and fatigue (66%), with visual changes, nausea and vomiting less frequently reported.[5,8] Symptoms relating to the specific hormonal deficiency may also be present, but patients may have biochemically low levels of pituitary hormones without symptoms.[15]

Biochemical tests. Hypophysitis results in deficiencies in all or some of the anterior pituitary hormones; in cases of suspected hypophysitis, testing of these hormones is recommended and should include TFTs (TSH, fT_3, fT_4), adrenal function tests (ACTH and cortisol), gonadal hormones (testosterone in men and estradiol in women), follicle-stimulating hormone (FSH) and LH. These tests should be performed at around 8 AM in the morning to obtain accurate levels.[4]

The anterior pituitary hormones most commonly deficient in cases of hypophysitis are the thyroid function hormones. The deficiency results in secondary hypothyroidism, which presents biochemically as a low or normal TSH level with low fT_4 and/or low T_3. Diagnosis of secondary hypothyoidism may be missed if fT_4 is not measured.[9] Secondary adrenal insufficiency is also common, causing low morning levels of ACTH and cortisol. Less frequently reported are deficiencies in the gonadal hormones (testosterone in men, estradiol in women) and the gonadotropins (FSH and LH). Panhypopituitarism (secondary hypothyroidism, secondary adrenal insufficiency, hypogonadotropic hypogonadism) can also occur.

Imaging. MRI of the sella should be performed when hypophysitis is suspected and before starting steroids. Pituitary enlargement and/or thickening of the pituitary stalk will occur in up to 75% of patients and can precede clinical or biochemical signs.[4] Although no abnormality will be demonstrated on MRI in 25% of patients, this is not a basis for excluding the diagnosis of hypophysitis.[8]

Primary adrenal insufficiency

Adrenal insufficiency, and the associated adrenal crisis, is a rare but potentially life-threatening irAE arising from ICI therapy. It has been reported in less than 3% of patients receiving combination therapy, with grade 3/4 events in 1.6% of patients and less than 1% of patients treated with anti-PD-1 monotherapy.[17]

Diagnostic evaluation will reveal electrolyte imbalances as well as abnormal adrenal biochemical tests (low morning cortisol and high ACTH) and evidence of volume depletion.

Physical examination. When primary adrenal insufficiency is suspected, a thorough head-to-toe assessment should be performed, with particular attention paid to potential causes of an adrenal crisis, such as evidence of infection.

Biochemical tests. Morning ACTH and cortisol levels must be assessed, as well as electrolytes. Evidence of primary insufficiency will be demonstrated biochemically by high levels of ACTH and low cortisol levels.

Imaging with adrenal CT could be considered to investigate possible metastases.

Type 1 diabetes

Type 1 diabetes mellitus is a rare endocrine irAE that has been reported in less than 1% of patients in clinical trials.[1,3,12] Many individuals present with diabetic ketoacidosis, while others have severe hyperglycemia. The use of high-dose corticosteroids to treat other irAEs or as supportive therapy for other cancer treatment may be a causative factor and should be considered.

Diagnostic evaluation for new or worsening type 1 diabetes should include a thorough clinical assessment for signs and symptoms such as polyuria and polydipsia, weight loss, nausea and vomiting. An extensive patient history should be taken that includes risk for diabetes[16] and recent corticosteroid therapy.

A blood glucose level should be measured at baseline and in the clinic before each ICI infusion and, if elevated blood glucose is found, patients should have fasting blood glucose measured. If type 1 diabetes is suspected, urinalysis for ketones should be performed and further testing for antibodies to insulin, glutamic acid decarboxylase (GAD) and islet cells should be considered.

When to refer

Management of endocrine toxicities can be challenging; referral to an endocrinologist is recommended in all cases of suspected or confirmed endocrinopathy. In particular, any patient with suspected or confirmed hypophysitis, primary adrenal insufficiency or type 1 diabetes should have their management overseen by an endocrinologist as they will need immediate hormone replacement and, often, acute inpatient management. As patients with confirmed endocrine toxicities from ICIs require life-long hormone replacement, management by an endocrinologist is warranted for long-term follow-up.

Management

Although grading of endocrinopathies according to the CTCAE[7] may not be sufficient as it does not always adequately incorporate symptoms with biochemical test results,[9] it provides a useful approach to management for patients with confirmed endocrine toxicity (Tables 8.6–8.10, pages 82–9).

Nursing considerations

Nurses should be aware that symptoms from endocrine toxicities are often vague and non-specific and can overlap with symptoms from advanced cancer and other treatments. They should therefore be alert to symptoms that may require further diagnostic evaluation,[18] as well as to overall trends in symptoms. Nurses who are administering ICIs should educate themselves on possible endocrine toxicities and associated symptoms as some endocrine irAEs differ from traditional cancer therapy toxicities and may not be familiar to oncology nurses.[6]

Nurses are instrumental in educating patients and carers about the various endocrinopathies, ensuring they are aware of clinical signs and symptoms, that treatment will require life-long hormone replacement and that completion of treatment will not resolve the toxicity. Nurses also have a key role in facilitating ongoing education, assessment and support as patients continue with ICI therapy following an endocrine toxicity.

Key points – endocrine-related adverse events

- Symptoms of endocrine toxicities can be vague and non-descript and may overlap with those of other conditions, such as advanced cancer, and therapies; health professionals should be aware of the symptoms that warrant further diagnostic evaluation.
- Baseline endocrine function should be undertaken before starting immune checkpoint inhibitor therapy to assist in the ongoing evaluation and diagnosis of possible endocrine toxicities.
- Diagnostic evaluation of endocrine toxicity must determine whether a hormone deficiency is primary or secondary, as this has treatment implications.
- All patients with a suspected or confirmed endocrinopathy should be referred to an endocrinologist to ensure optimal long-term follow-up and management.
- Even after completion of therapy, the toxicity does not resolve; patients need to be advised that they will require life-long hormone replacement, but they should be reassured that they can maintain a good quality of life.

Key references

1. Eigentler TK, Hassel JC, Berking C et al. Diagnosis, monitoring and management of immune-related adverse drug reactions of anti-PD-1 antibody therapy. *Cancer Treat Rev* 2016;45:7–18.

2. Bertrand A, Kostine M, Barnetche T et al. Immune related adverse events associated with anti-CTLA-4 antibodies: systematic review and meta-analysis. *BMC Med* 2015;13:211.

3. Sznol M, Ferrucci PF, Hogg D et al. Pooled analysis safety profile of nivolumab and ipilimumab combination therapy in patients with advanced melanoma. *J Clin Oncol* 2017;35:3815–22.

4. Kottschade L, Brys A, Peikert T et al. A multidisciplinary approach to toxicity management of modern immune checkpoint inhibitors in cancer therapy. *Melanoma Res* 2016;26:469–80.

5. Puzanov I, Diab A, Abdallah K et al. Managing toxicities associated with immune checkpoint inhibitors: consensus recommendations from the Society for Immunotherapy of Cancer (SITC) Toxicity Management Working Group. *J Immunother Cancer* 2017;5:95.

6. McGettigan S, Rubin KM. PD-1 inhibitor therapy. *Clin J Oncol Nurs* 2017;21(suppl):42–51.

7. National Institutes of Health, National Cancer Institute. Common Terminology Criteria for Adverse Events (CTCAE) v.5, November 2017. https://ctep.cancer.gov/protocoldevelopment/electronic_applications/docs/CTCAE_v5_Quick_Reference_8.5x11.pdf, last accessed 2 April 2019.

8. Dadu R, Zobniw C, Diab A. Managing adverse events with immune checkpoint agents. *Cancer J* 2016;22:121–9.

9. Illouz F, Briet C, Cloix L et al. Endocrine toxicity of immune checkpoint inhibitors: essential crosstalk between endocrinologists and oncologists. *Cancer Med* 2017;6:1923–9.

10. Postow M, Chesney J, Pavlick A et al. Nivolumab and ipilimumab versus ipilimumab in untreated melanoma. *N Engl J Med* 2015;372:2006–17.

11. Weber JS, Hodi FS, Wolchok JD et al. Safety profile of nivolumab monotherapy: a pooled analysis of patients with advanced melanoma. *J Clin Oncol* 2017;35:785–91.

12. Davies M, Duffield EA. Safety of checkpoint inhibitors for cancer treatment: strategies for patient monitoring and management of immune-mediated adverse events. *Immunotargets Ther* 2017;6:51–71.

13. Nagai H, Muto M. Optimal management of immune-related adverse events resulting from treatment with immune checkpoint inhibitors: a review and update. *Int J Clin Oncol* 2018;23:410–20.

14. Morganstein DL, Lai Z, Spain L et al. Thyroid abnormalities following the use of cytotoxic T-lymphocyte antigen-4 and programmed death receptor protein-1 inhibitors in the treatment of melanoma. *Clin Endocrinol* 2017;86:614–20.

15. Michot JM, Bigenwald C, Champiat S et al. Immune-related adverse events with immune checkpoint blockade: a comprehensive review. *Eur J Cancer* 2016;54:139–48.

16. Brahmer JR, Lacchetti C, Schneider BJ et al. Management of immune-related adverse events in patients treated with immune checkpoint inhibitor therapy: American Society of Clinical Oncology Clinical Practice Guideline. *J Clin Oncol* 2018;36:1714–68.

17. Sznol M, Postow MA, Davies MJ et al. Endocrine-related adverse events associated with immune checkpoint blockade and expert insights on their management. *Cancer Treat Rev* 2017;58:70–6.

18. Madden KM, Hoffner B. Ipilimumab-based therapy: consensus statement from the Faculty of the Melanoma Nursing Initiative on managing adverse events with ipilimumab monotherapy and combination therapy with nivolumab. *Clin J Oncol Nurs* 2017;21(suppl):30–41.

5

Pulmonary adverse events

Pulmonary toxicity from immune checkpoint inhibitors (ICIs), most significantly immune-related pneumonitis, while uncommon, is one of the most serious adverse events associated with ICIs, with deaths relating to pneumonitis reported in a number of clinical studies.[1]

Pneumonitis

Pneumonitis is more commonly reported with anti-programmed cell death 1 (PD-1) or anti-programmed death ligand 1 (PD-L1) therapies than with anti-cytotoxic T lymphocyte-associated antigen 4 (CTLA-4) monotherapy or combination (anti-CTLA-4/anti-PD-1) regimens, occurring in 0–10.6%, less than 1% and 6.6% of patients, respectively.[1-3] Pneumonitis may be less likely to resolve in patients treated with combination therapy compared with monotherapy.[4] Grade 3/4 events have been reported in less than 5% of patients treated with anti-PD-1/PD-L1 monotherapy and less than 2% of those receiving combination ICI therapy.[1,5] Grading definitions for pneumonitis are shown in Table 8.11 (page 90).

Immune-related pneumonitis of any grade more commonly affects patients with a diagnosis of lung cancer than any other cancer patient,[1] though it is unclear why this association exists. It may be that these patients are more likely to have: pre-existing pulmonary conditions arising from tobacco exposure; previous thoracic radiotherapy; and/or previous exposure to drugs associated with lung toxicity, such as gemcitabine and tyrosine kinase inhibitors.[1,5] However, immune-related pneumonitis has been demonstrated in both former and current smokers (56%) as well as never smokers (44%).[3] Pneumonitis with ICI treatment does not appear to be more common in patients with lung cancer who have already undergone thoracic radiotherapy than those who have not had radiotherapy.[6]

Onset. The median time to onset of pneumonitis is approximately 3 months,[3] but wide variations in the timing have been reported.

It seems to start earlier in patients treated with combination therapy than in those receiving monotherapy.[3,4]

Diagnostic evaluation of immune-related pneumonitis is often reached through clinical assessment and radiological investigation; however, for some patients, radiological evidence may appear before clinical signs develop, while others may remain asymptomatic despite evidence of pneumonitis on CT.[5,7]

Clinical presentation. Symptoms of pneumonitis include dyspnea, dry cough, wheeze, reduced exercise tolerance and, less commonly, fever and chest pain.[7,8] Hypoxia can occur and may progress rapidly, leading to respiratory failure.[5,8] A full patient history should be taken to determine changes in respiratory function from baseline and pulse oximetry performed, both at rest and with exercise.

Imaging. For patients where pneumonitis is suspected, high-resolution CT should be urgently performed, as chest X-ray is an insufficiently accurate tool for diagnostic evaluation, failing to identify ~25% of cases.[5] The radiological appearance of pneumonitis varies. Most commonly, pneumonitis manifests radiologically as ground-glass opacities, patchy nodular infiltrates or similar to cryptogenic organizing pneumonia. It can also present with patterns similar to non-specific interstitial pneumonitis, hypersensitivity, acute interstitial pneumonia and acute respiratory distress syndrome.[2,3,5,7] Examples of radiological subtypes are shown in Figure 5.1.

Other tests. Lung biopsy is not usually necessary to confirm diagnosis where clinical and radiological signs are consistent with pneumonitis; however, a bronchoscopy should be considered to exclude differentials such as infection in patients with grade 2 pneumonitis or higher, and lung function testing should also be considered for these patients.[8,9]

Management. For all grades of pneumonitis, the mainstay of treatment is stopping the ICI therapy. In cases of grade 1 pneumonitis, therapy should be stopped, with close monitoring for symptoms every 2–3 days and repeat imaging at least every 3 weeks or before the next scheduled dose of ICI therapy (whichever occurs first) to ensure pulmonary infiltrates have resolved.[5,7] Rechallenging patients with ICI

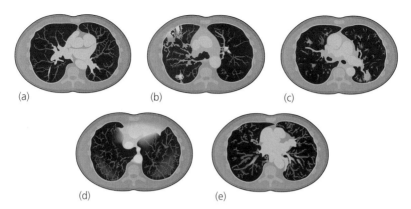

Figure 5.1 Examples of radiological subtypes of pneumonitis seen in patients treated with immune checkpoint inhibitors: (a) ground glass opacities; (b) cryptogenic organizing pneumonia-like; (c) pneumonitis not otherwise specified; (d) hypersensitivity; and (e) interstitial with discrete areas of attenuation.

therapy following resolution and with close follow-up of symptoms is appropriate.

Patients with grade 1 pneumonitis may be managed as outpatients, but in most cases of grade 2 and all cases of grade 3/4 toxicity, admission to hospital for management is recommended.[7,10] Management is with immunosuppressive agents (Table 8.11, page 90).

Sarcoidosis

Sarcoidosis is another pulmonary toxicity that has been associated with ICI therapy. Case studies within the literature report sarcoidosis predominantly in patients treated with anti-PD-1/PD-L1 and anti-CTLA-4 monotherapies, but it has also been associated with combination ICI therapy.[11]

Diagnostic evaluation. Clinical presentation of sarcoidosis is diverse and patients may be asymptomatic or present with a cough, wheeze, fatigue and chest pain. Chest imaging should be performed; evidence of intrathoracic lymphadenopathy is suggestive of pulmonary sarcoidosis. However, as radiological and clinical findings can mimic disease progression, a biopsy to confirm diagnosis – considered the gold standard – should be performed.[7,8,11,12]

Once diagnosis is confirmed, patients should undergo an ECG and eye examination to investigate the involvement of other organs.[7,12]

Management. Currently, there are no guidelines for the management of pulmonary sarcoidosis specifically arising from ICI use; management is based on standard management guidelines for sarcoidosis in the general population (Table 8.12, page 92). There are no formal Common Terminology Criteria for Adverse Events (CTCAE) grading criteria for sarcoidosis, but management differs according to severity.[12]

Once a diagnosis is confirmed, ICI therapy should be stopped. Baseline pulmonary function tests should be performed along with baseline CT and frequent monitoring of resting oxygen saturation. Patients with persistent pulmonary symptoms, a decline in lung function, progressive radiological changes or hypercalcemia should be treated according to standard guidelines.[7,13]

Differential diagnosis

Immune-related pneumonitis should be considered when any patient receiving an ICI presents with new or worsening respiratory symptoms; however, a number of differential diagnoses should be considered and excluded during initial work-up (Table 5.1). Referral to

TABLE 5.1

Differential diagnosis for immune-related pneumonitis

Infective causes	Other
Typical	• Interstitial inflammation from other drugs
• Pneumonia	
• Tuberculosis	• Inhaled irritants
• Fungal infection	• Radiation pneumonitis, if patient has had thoracic radiotherapy in preceding 3 months
• *Pneumocystis jirovecii*	
• Cytomegalovirus	
Atypical	• Pulmonary involvement of malignancy
• *Legionella pneumophila*	
• Chlamydia	

Sources: Dadu et al. 2016; Michot et al. 2016; and Eigentler et al. 2016.[10,14,15]

a respiratory specialist to facilitate bronchoscopy and to an infectious disease specialist should be initiated.[10,14,15]

The incidence of pneumonitis is higher in patients undergoing radiation therapy. The cause (radiation vs ICI) should be identified as it may have implications for ongoing treatment.[16]

When to refer

All patients with clinical or radiological evidence of pneumonitis should be referred to a respiratory specialist to facilitate bronchoscopy. In cases of grade 2 or higher pneumonitis, referral to an infectious disease consultant should be considered. Patients with pneumonitis often require long-term follow-up, which should be managed by a respiratory specialist.

Nursing considerations

Nurses play a key role in the education, assessment and management of patients with suspected or confirmed pneumonitis from ICI therapy. Nurses should explain the signs and symptoms of pneumonitis when providing pretreatment information to patients and carers. It is important that they explain clearly to patients when to get in touch with their healthcare team.

Nurses should perform a baseline assessment of patients before ICI treatment starts, documenting a patient's usual respiratory function, so that any changes such as new or worsening cough, dyspnea or wheeze can be identified when repeat assessment is carried out before the next infusion. Nurses should also monitor pulse oxygen saturations at each visit. If a patient at a recent visit reported being able to walk on an incline but is now unable to do so, it is the inconsistency with the pretreatment assessment by the nurse that will alert the healthcare team to possible symptoms that require further diagnosic evaluation. This is particularly important for patients with lung cancer, who may have respiratory symptoms from their disease, and those who have underlying pulmonary disease such as chronic obstructive pulmonary disease, interstitial lung disease or pulmonary fibrosis. By being aware of the patient's baseline respiratory status, nurses are able to quickly detect changes that may indicate immune-related pneumonitis. This is crucial, as failure to detect symptoms early may result in delayed diagnosis and poor clinical outcomes.

For patients with grade 1 pneumonitis who are being managed as an outpatient, nurses have an important role in monitoring for worsening symptoms and ensuring that care is escalated quickly when appropriate. In addition, for those patients who are slowly tapering steroids over 4–6 weeks, nurses can provide ongoing support and monitoring so that any changes or deterioration of symptoms during this time are identified early.

Key points – pulmonary adverse events

- Pneumonitis is an uncommon but serious adverse event from immune checkpoint inhibitor (ICI) therapy that has been associated with treatment-related deaths; the incidence is higher in patients using anti-programmed cell death 1 (PD-1)/programmed cell death ligand 1 (PD-L1) therapy, those with lung cancer and those who have had radiation therapy.
- The differential diagnoses for pneumonitis include infective etiologies and pulmonary progression of disease.
- The mainstay of treatment is the cessation of the ICI and immunosuppressive agents; patients with grade 2 or higher pneumonitis should be admitted to hospital for management.
- All patients with clinical and radiological signs of pneumonitis should be referred to a respiratory specialist; referral to an infectious disease specialist should be considered for patients with grade 2 or higher pneumonitis.
- Nurses have a key role in knowing patients' baseline respiratory state so that subtle changes may be identified; they can also educate patients and carers about the signs and symptoms of pneumonitis.

Key references

1. Nishino M, Giobbie-Hurder A, Hatabu H et al. Incidence of programmed cell death 1 inhibitor-related pneumonitis in patients with advanced cancer. A systematic review and meta-analysis. *JAMA Oncol* 2016;2:1607–16.

2. Naidoo J, Page DB, Li BT et al. Toxicities of the anti-PD-1 and anti-PD-L1 immune checkpoint antibodies. *Ann Oncol* 2015;26: 2375–91.

3. Naidoo J, Wang X, Woo K et al. Pneumonitis in patients treated with anti-programmed death-1/ programmed death ligand 1 therapy. *J Clin Oncol* 2017;35:709–17.

4. Postow M, Chesney J, Pavlick A et al. Nivolumab and ipilimumab versus ipilimumab in untreated melanoma. *N Engl J Med* 2015;372:2006–17.

5. Chuzi S, Tavora F, Cruz M et al. Clinical features, diagnostic challenges, and management strategies in checkpoint inhibitor related pneumonitis. *Cancer Manag Res* 2017;9:207–13.

6. Hwang WL, Niemierko A, Hwang KL et al. Clinical outcomes in patients with metastatic lung cancer treated with PD-1/PD-L1 inhibitors and thoracic radiotherapy. *JAMA Oncol* 2018;4:253–5.

7. Puzanov I, Diab A, Abdallah K et al. Managing toxicities associated with immune checkpoint inhibitors: consensus recommendations from the Society for Immunotherapy of Cancer (SITC) Toxicity Management Working Group. *J Immunother Cancer* 2017;5:95.

8. Brahmer JR, Lacchetti C, Schneider BJ et al. Management of immune-related adverse events in patients treated with immune checkpoint inhibitor therapy: American Society of Clinical Oncology Clinical Practice Guideline. *J Clin Oncol* 2018;36:1714–68.

9. Kottschade L, Brys A, Peikert T et al. A multidisciplinary approach to toxicity management of modern immune checkpoint inhibitors in cancer therapy. *Melanoma Res* 2016;26: 469–80.

10. Dadu R, Zobniw C, Diab A. Managing adverse events with immune checkpoint agents. *Cancer J* 2016;22:121–9.

11. Reuss JE, Kunk PR, Stowman AM et al. Sarcoidosis in the setting of combination ipilimumab and nivolumab immunotherapy: a case report and review of the literature. *J Immunother Cancer* 2016;4:94.

12. National Institutes of Health, National Cancer Institute. Common Terminology Criteria for Adverse Events (CTCAE) v.5, November 2017. https://ctep.cancer.gov/ protocoldevelopment/electronic_ applications/docs/CTCAE_v5_Quick_ Reference_8.5x11.pdf, last accessed 2 April 2019.

13. Winer A, Bodor JN, Borghaei H. Identifying and managing the adverse effects of immune checkpoint blockade. *J Thorac Dis* 2018;10(suppl 3):480–9.

14. Michot JM, Bigenwald C, Champiat S et al. Immune-related adverse events with immune checkpoint blockade: a comprehensive review. *Eur J Cancer* 2016;54:139–48.

15. Eigentler TK, Hassel JC, Berking C et al. Diagnosis, monitoring and management of immune-related adverse drug reactions of anti-PD-1 antibody therapy. *Cancer Treat Rev* 2016;45:7–18.

16. Antonia SJ, Villegas A, Daniel D et al. Durvalumab after chemoradiotherapy in stage III non-small-cell lung cancer. *N Engl J Med* 2017;377:1919–29.

6 Less frequent adverse events

As the use of immune checkpoint inhibitors (ICIs) and clinical experience have increased, so has the spectrum of immune-related adverse events (irAEs), with a number of rare toxicities being attributed to ICI therapy. While incidence is low, these rare irAEs can be serious and deaths have been reported.

Renal toxicity

Renal toxicity is a rare complication of ICI therapy; it has been reported in less than 5% of patients receiving combination (anti-cytotoxic T lymphocyte-associated antigen 4 [CTLA-4]/anti-programmed cell death 1 [PD-1]) regimens and less than 3% of patients treated with single-agent CTLA-4 or PD-1 monoclonal antibody (mAb) (any grade).[1-3] Grade 3/4 renal toxicity has been reported in less than 1% of monotherapy-treated patients and 1.6% of patients treated with combination therapy.[2,3] However, a review suggests that renal irAEs may be under-reported and the incidence could be as high as ~29%.[4]

Interstitial nephritis is the most common cause of acute kidney injury (AKI) in patients who have received ICIs, but cases of lupus nephritis and granulomatous nephritis have also been reported.[5,6] Time to onset of AKI varies; it has been reported after 2–3 months of treatment with CTLA-4-specific antibodies and 3–10 months following anti-PD-1 therapy.[1,5,6]

Diagnostic evaluation. Immune-related nephritis should be considered in ICI-treated patients who present with impaired renal function. Initial work-up should, however, exclude other causes, such as concomitant medications, infection, urinary tract obstruction and hypovolemia.[5,7] Serum creatinine, urea and electrolytes should be monitored before starting immunotherapy and then before each ICI infusion. In patients with elevated creatinine (grade 1, creatinine ×1.5–2.0 over baseline),[8] monitoring should increase to weekly bloods; in cases of suspected grade 2 renal toxicity (creatinine ×2–3 over baseline),[8] serum creatinine should be monitored every 2–3 days.[5] Urinalysis does not need to be performed other than to eliminate urinary tract infection as a possible cause. Immunosuppressive therapy should not be delayed to perform a biopsy when there is no alternative etiology.

When to refer. A nephrology consultation should be sought for patients with an elevated creatinine consistent with grade 2 toxicity or higher. Patients with any evidence of renal failure should also be urgently referred.

Management. As with other irAEs from ICI therapy, management is algorithm driven and based on the toxicity grade (Table 8.13, page 93). Treatment should be stopped in cases of grade 1 toxicity while other etiologies are excluded and in all cases of grade 2 toxicity or higher.

Musculoskeletal toxicities

Musculoskeletal and rheumatic toxicities can provide a diagnostic challenge. The high prevalence of musculoskeletal problems in the general population means that they may be under-reported in association with ICI therapy. Symptoms such as arthralgia and myalgia have been reported in 2–12% of patients receiving ICI therapy, most commonly in patients treated with PD-1-specific antibodies or combination therapy, but they do not always represent a rheumatic irAE, such as inflammatory arthritis.[2,7,9-11] The most frequently reported rheumatic irAEs are inflammatory arthritis, polymyalgia-like syndromes and myositis. Patients may present with oligo- or polyarthritis that affects large and/or small joints.

The time to onset for musculoskeletal irAEs is typically many months after starting ICI therapy and they can persist beyond treatment discontinuation.

Diagnostic evaluation of any suspected musculoskeletal irAEs should begin with a complete history and examination. The patient's joints should be evaluated for signs of swelling and pain, with testing for range of motion and muscle strength. Blood tests should include antinuclear antibody, rheumatoid factor and inflammatory markers such as erythrocyte sedimentation rate and C-reactive protein.

For patients with suspected myositis, additional tests should be performed, including creatine kinase, alanine transaminase/aspartate transaminase and lactate dehydrogenase, as well as troponin to evaluate myocardial involvement and an ECG.[2]

In cases of inflammatory arthritis not responsive to treatment, ultrasound or MRI of the affected joints could be considered.[9]

When to refer. Patients with symptoms consistent with grade 2 toxicity or higher should be referred to a rheumatologist, as should those with symptoms persisting for 6 weeks or more. All cases of suspected or confirmed myositis should be referred to a rheumatologist or neurologist.

Management of musculoskeletal events is summarized in Tables 8.14–8.16 (pages 94–6).

Neurological toxicities

Neurological toxicities associated with ICI therapy have an overall incidence ranging from 3.8% in patients receiving anti-CTLA-4 monotherapy to 6.1% with anti-PD-1 monotherapy.[12] As with other toxicities, incidence is higher with combination anti-CTLA-4/anti-PD-1 therapy, with the reported incidence reaching 12%.[12] Grade 3/4 toxicity has been reported in less than 1% of patients, regardless of mAb.[2]

Reported neurological events include myasthenia gravis, aseptic meningitis, encephalitis, sensory motor neuropathy such as Guillain–Barré syndrome, mononeuritis multiplex and transverse myelitis. The timing of onset of neurological toxicity varies from 6 to 13 weeks.

Diagnostic evaluation. Initial steps in the diagnostic evaluation of neurological toxicity should be to rule out central nervous system progression of the underlying cancer as well as infective or metabolic etiologies. Clinical evaluation for symptoms such as headache, confusion, memory or behavior changes and seizure activity should also be carried out.

MRI of the brain (with and without contrast) should be performed, as well as cerebrospinal fluid evaluation to rule out leptomeningeal disease, autoimmune encephalitis and aseptic meningitis.

For suspected cases of Guillain–Barré syndrome, a lumbar puncture and nerve conduction studies should be considered. Possible paraneoplastic phenomena should be excluded during diagnostic evaluation.

When to refer. All patients with suspected or confirmed neurological toxicity, especially those with grade 2 or higher symptoms, should be referred to a neurologist for assessment.

Management of neurological irAEs is guided by the findings of diagnostic evaluation but, as with other AEs, management is algorithm driven and determined by severity of the toxicity. For grade 1 conditions, ICI therapy can be continued, but with close monitoring for escalating symptoms. In cases of grade 2 symptoms or higher, ICI therapy should be stopped until a diagnosis has been determined; therapy should be restarted in consultation with a neurologist. Prednisone, 0.5–1 mg/kg, or methylprednisolone, at a dose between 1 and 4 mg/kg, should be started in cases of grade 2 toxicity or higher. Additional management, including plasmapheresis or intravenous immunoglobulin, may be indicated.

Ophthalmologic toxicities

Ocular irAEs are reported in up to 1% of patients treated with anti-PD-1/programmed cell death ligand 1 (PD-L1) and anti-CTLA-4 monotherapies as well as those treated with combination therapy.[2,6,13,14] While the incidence is low, the most common ocular irAE reported is uveitis, but cases of blepharitis, episcleritis, keratitis and optic nerve swelling have also been reported.[5]

Diagnostic evaluation. Patients should be told to report, promptly, any new symptoms such as blurred vision, floaters, changes in color vision, redness, photophobia or light sensitivity, visual field changes or double vision. Initial diagnostic evaluation should include examination of visual acuity, penlight inspection of the anterior part of the eye and testing pupils for equal reaction.

When to refer. All patients with suspected ocular toxicity from ICIs should be referred to an ophthalmologist for consultation, evaluation and diagnosis. Additional tests may be warranted that require ophthalmology access. Urgent referral to an ophthalmologist is necessary for any suspected grade 3/4 toxicity.

Management is summarized in Tables 8.17–8.19 (pages 97–9).

Cardiovascular toxicity

Cardiovascular toxicity, while rare – having been reported in less than 0.1% of patients receiving ICI therapy – is one of the most serious irAEs and often results in death. Cardiovascular toxicity has been reported with all ICI antibodies and is slightly higher in patients treated with combination therapy (0.27%).[7] The median time to onset is 10 weeks after treatment initiation, but it can start as early as 2 weeks and can be as delayed as 32 weeks following treatment initiation.[15] Cardiovascular toxicities that have been reported include myocarditis, myocardial fibrosis, cardiomyopathy and conduction abnormalities.

Diagnostic evaluation should begin with a clinical assessment to identify symptoms such as chest pain, shortness of breath, peripheral edema, fatigue, palpitations and arrhythmias. Other etiologies such as a pulmonary embolism or pneumonitis should be considered and excluded. An ECG should be performed; bloods tests should include troponin levels as well as CK. Further tests such as stress tests or cardiac MRI can also be considered where indicated. For patients with suspected or confirmed myocarditis, an endomyocardial biopsy should be considered.

When to refer. Patients with suspected or confirmed cardiovascular toxicity should be referred to a cardiologist for diagnostic evaluation and diagnosis. Any patient with abnormal cardiac tests should be referred urgently. For patients with suspected or confirmed myocarditis, admission to hospital is warranted.

Management. For all grades, it is recommended that the patient stops ICI therapy (Table 8.20, page 99). In cases of grade 2/3 toxicity, management with systemic corticosteroids (1–2 mg/kg/day) is indicated, with escalation of dosing in those patients with confirmed grade 3/4 toxicity or patients who do not respond to initial management. Escalation to additional immunosuppressive agents such as infliximab, mycophenolate mofetil or antithymocyte globulin may also be considered in this latter patient group.[2,7]

Hematologic toxicity

Hematologic irAEs from ICI therapy are rare, but reported cases include anemia, thrombocytopenia, neutropenia, myelodysplasia and hemophilia.[5] Cytopenia may be more frequent with lymphoma than with solid tumors.[14]

Diagnostic evaluation should exclude hematologic causes of cytopenia, such as bone marrow infiltration of malignancy.[14] A complete blood count should be performed at baseline before starting ICI therapy and before each treatment. Other etiologies should be excluded, such as gastrointestinal bleeding, disease progression or other medications. A bone marrow biopsy should be considered if the cause cannot be identified.

When to refer. A hematologist referral should be considered for all patients who present with cytopenia if no other etiology has been identified.

Management. In cases of low-grade hematologic irAEs, treatment with ICIs may continue, with close monitoring. In more severe cases, corticosteroids should be started. Additional supportive therapy should be initiated if indicated by the presenting irAE.

Key points – less frequent adverse events

- Rare immune-related adverse events (irAEs) from immune checkpoint inhibitor therapy can be missed, but they are often serious and have been associated with treatment-related deaths.
- Referral to appropriate specialists is necessary as oncologists are not experienced in treating these rare irAEs.
- The spectrum of rheumatologic, neurological, cardiovascular and hematologic irAEs is wide and while management includes corticosteroid use, it is often based on established guidelines; patients should, therefore, be managed in consultation with a specialist.
- Nurses must be aware of the potential for rare irAEs so that they do not overlook signs during patient assessment.

Key references

1. Eigentler TK, Hassel JC, Berking C et al. Diagnosis, monitoring and management of immune-related adverse drug reactions of anti-PD-1 antibody therapy. Cancer Treat Rev 2016; 45:7–18.

2. Brahmer JR, Lacchetti C, Schneider BJ et al. Management of immune-related adverse events in patients treated with immune checkpoint inhibitor therapy: American Society of Clinical Oncology Clinical Practice Guideline. J Clin Oncol 2018;36:1714–68.

3. Sznol M, Ferrucci PF, Hogg D et al. Pooled analysis safety profile of nivolumab and ipilimumab combination therapy in patients with advanced melanoma. J Clin Oncol 2017;35:3815–22.

4. Wanchoo R, Karam S, Uppal NN et al. Adverse renal effects of immune checkpoint inhibitors: a narrative review. Am J Nephrol 2017;45:160–9.

5. Puzanov I, Diab A, Abdallah K et al. Managing toxicities associated with immune checkpoint inhibitors: consensus recommendations from the Society for Immunotherapy of Cancer (SITC) Toxicity Management Working Group. J Immunother Cancer 2017;5:95.

6. Naidoo J, Page DB, Li BT et al. Toxicities of the anti-PD-1 and anti-PD-L1 immune checkpoint antibodies. Ann Oncol 2015;26: 2375–91.

7. Haanen JBAG, Carbonnel F, Robert C et al. Management of toxicities from immunotherapy: ESMO Clinical Practice Guidelines for diagnosis, treatment and follow-up. Ann Oncol 2017;28(suppl 4):iv119–42.

8. National Institutes of Health, National Cancer Institute. Common Terminology Criteria for Adverse Events (CTCAE) v.5, November 2017. https://ctep.cancer.gov/protocoldevelopment/electronic_applications/docs/CTCAE_v5_Quick_Reference_8.5x11.pdf, last accessed 2 April 2019.

9. Naidoo J, Cappelli LC, Forde PM et al. Inflammatory arthritis: a newly recognized adverse event of immune checkpoint blockade. *Oncologist* 2017;22:627–30.

10. Weber JS, Hodi FS, Wolchok JD et al. Safety profile of nivolumab monotherapy: a pooled analysis of patients with advanced melanoma. *J Clin Oncol* 2017;35:785–91.

11. Postow MA, Chesney J, Pavlick AC et al. Nivolumb and ipilimumab versus ipilimumab in untreated melanoma. *N Engl J Med* 2015;372:2006–17.

12. Cuzzubbo S, Javeri F, Tissier M et al. Neurological adverse events associated with immune-checkpoint inhibitors: review of the literature. *Eur J Cancer* 2017;73:1–8.

13. Winer A, Bodor JN, Borghaei H. Identifying and managing the adverse effects of immune checkpoint blockade. *J Thorac Dis* 2018;10(suppl 3):480–9.

14. Michot JM, Bigenwald C, Champiat S et al. Immune-related adverse events with immune checkpoint blockade: a comprehensive review. *Eur J Cancer* 2016;54:139–48.

15. Jain V, Bahia J, Mohebtash M et al. Cardiovascular complications associated with novel cancer immunotherapies. *Curr Treat Options Cardiovascular Med* 2017;19:36.

7 Optimizing patient care and early recognition of immune-related adverse events

Emergency department involvement

As the use of immune checkpoint inhibitors (ICIs) becomes more widespread, and ICIs become increasingly used in combination with other therapies, so the incidence and spectrum of immune-related adverse events (irAEs) will increase. Many patients will present to the emergency department (ED) with acute symptoms. Physicians in the ED are familiar with management strategies for chemotherapy-associated toxicity and, when patients present with a fever, an algorithm response is triggered that is guided by established protocol. However, irAEs related to ICI use are not so familiar and risk being overlooked, with the etiology attributed to infection or disease.[1] Emergency physicians have a significant role in ensuring irAEs are identified and investigated early and that prompt immunosuppressive therapy is started to avoid complications and escalation of symptoms, decrease associated morbidity and mortality and enable patients to continue on ICI therapy.[2]

Engagement with the ED team is essential to raise awareness of the potential for irAEs from ICIs and the associated management algorithms. It is also necessary to ensure that a suspected or confirmed irAE is communicated to the treating oncologist so they may guide management in consultation with organ-specific specialist physicians.

To help ED physicians identify patients using ICIs so that irAEs are included in the differential diagnosis, it is useful if patients carry an immunotherapy drug safety card in their wallets that states the therapy the patient is receiving. In addition, using electronic medical records as a mechanism to alert ED staff that a patient is being treated with an ICI can assist in early identification and management.[2,3]

Multidisciplinary teams

Adverse events from ICIs have the potential to affect any organ and therefore the spectrum of potential toxicity is diverse. As the use of

ICIs increases, so does the likelihood of both common and rarer irAEs. Many oncologists are not familiar or comfortable with the clinical management of these and do not have the necessary experience to manage ICI toxicities effectively.[4] A multidisciplinary approach to management, with early engagement and consultation with organ-specific specialists, is therefore essential. Furthermore, referral to specialists such as gastroenterologists or respiratory specialists is often necessary to facilitate diagnostic work-up with procedures such as flexible sigmoidoscopy or bronchoscopy and to enable access to immunosuppressive agents such as infliximab.

Engaging with departments to identify organ-specific specialists who have an interest in the management of irAEs can be beneficial. Not only does it allow organ-specific physicians to gain experience and increase their knowledge of the management of toxicities, it ensures optimal management as referral pathways are established.

Patient education

Comprehensive education should be provided to patients and their carers before ICI therapy is started. As an immune response can occur even after treatment has ended, key information should be reiterated throughout treatment and once treatment has concluded. It must be emphasized to patients, especially those who have previously been treated with chemotherapy, that the mechanism of action of ICIs differs from traditional chemotherapy, as does the corresponding side-effect profile.

Patient information should cover the mechanism of ICI action, possible patterns and timings of response and information about possible irAEs, including:

- signs and symptoms of immune-related toxicities
- the importance of reporting symptoms early to allow prompt management
- who to report to within the healthcare team
- when to present to the ED (Table 7.1)
- how irAEs are managed
- the possibility of referral to other specialists to assist with management
- the need for life-long hormone replacement if the patient develops an endocrine toxicity.

TABLE 7.1

Signs that need immediate medical attention/emergency department presentation

- Blood or mucus in the stool
- Jaundice
- Skin blisters
- Chest pain
- Oliguria or hematuria
- Any neurological symptoms

It is important that patients and carers are given enough information so that they have the knowledge to identify signs and symptoms but are not overwhelmed, which is why it is essential that education is continuous and ongoing throughout treatment. Common irAEs should be highlighted, but it is important that patients are aware of the possibility of rarer toxicities so that they do not dismiss symptoms.

Patients and carers must be reassured that, in most cases, irAEs can be managed with treatment interruption and steroids if identified early. In cases when symptoms are vague and non-descript, patients should be told that it is vital that they contact the healthcare team to inform them of changes in their health.

Educational resources to support the understanding of irAEs should be tailored to the individual patient/carer, with consideration given to the individual's level of health literacy. A multimodal approach should be adopted, with printed materials, group education sessions (with videos and/or presentations) and online educational resources.[3]

A toxicity checklist can be useful to help patients recognize symptoms. If the nurse uses a toxicity checklist before each infusion, it helps patients by highlighting the common signs and symptoms of irAEs. Such a checklist should include the elements shown in Figure 7.1.

Clinical assessment

Assess the patient for treatment-related side effects and grade the following toxicities according to the CTCAE grading: 0 – nil, 1 – mild, 2 – moderate, 3 – severe, 4 – life threatening. See pages 3–4 for more information.

Date					
Gastrointestinal and hepatotoxicity					
Mucositis oral (mouth ulcers)					
Diarrhea					
Abdominal pain					

Gastrointestinal and hepatotoxicity

- Mucositis oral (mouth ulcers)
- Diarrhea
- Abdominal pain
- Mucus and/or blood present in stools
- Jaundice
- Nausea
- Vomiting
- Changes to urine color
- Bruising (more often than normal)
- Anorexia (loss of appetite)

Skin

- Pruritus
- Rash
- Peeling
- Blistering

Pulmonary

- Dyspnea (difficult or labored breathing)
- New or worsening cough
- Chest pain

Renal toxicity

- Hematuria
- Reduced urine output (oliguria)
- Back pain
- Swollen legs, ankles or feet

Neurological

- Paresthesia (tingling or numb feet and hands)
- Facial weakness
- Left- and/or right-sided weakness (e.g. arms, legs)
- Headache
- Photophobia (eye sensitivity to light)
- Ataxia (balance and gait changes)
- Cognitive changes (mood, judgment, perception)
- Memory impairment

Endocrine (headache may also indicate endocrine toxicity)

- Chills
- Fever
- Fatigue
- Increased sensitivity to heat or cold
- Blurred vision
- Excessive thirst
- Excessive urination

Figure 7.1 A toxicity checklist that is completed at baseline and before each infusion supports discussions with patients about potential events and facilitates effective tracking of health changes.

Nursing considerations

Nurses have a critical role in the care and management of patients using ICIs. They are often the first and primary contact for patients and carers and therefore have a vital role in ensuring the prompt identification and management of irAEs. The role of the nurse for patients on ICIs encompasses education, assessment, coordination, monitoring and support.

It is often nurses who provide education before treatment starts and therefore they are ideally positioned to ensure patients and carers have an in-depth understanding of possible AEs and to provide additional explanation and support. Nurses will also provide ongoing and continuous education to patients and carers throughout treatment.

In most centers, pretreatment patient assessment is undertaken by nurses. Nurses are therefore key to ensuring that signs and symptoms of suspected irAEs requiring further diagnostic evaluation are identified early. Assessment should be undertaken using an ICI-specific tool (see Figure 7.1), which will:

- ensure appropriate questions are asked of the patient to detect signs and symptoms of irAEs
- facilitate correct grading of toxicity so that care is quickly escalated and management algorithms can be followed
- standardize assessment
- allow symptom trends to be identified.

Advanced practice nurses have an important role in the assessment of patients when escalation of care and further diagnostic evaluation is required for suspected irAEs. Advanced practice nurses also have a pivotal role in monitoring patients with suspected irAEs through regular communication to assess symptoms so that changes can be identified quickly and care escalated.

For patients who have been treated for a confirmed irAE, nurses can provide monitoring and support when tapering corticosteroids. The nurse can regularly follow-up with the patient and/or carer to ensure steroids are being tapered appropriately and can promptly identify and escalate a symptom flare.

Management of patients with a confirmed irAE requires a multidisciplinary approach, often with multiple specialists. Nurses can assist in the coordination of care across multiple specialties to ensure effective and timely management.

Patients with pre-existing autoimmune conditions

Patients with pre-existing autoimmune conditions, such as ulcerative colitis, Crohn's disease or rheumatoid arthritis, have traditionally been excluded from clinical trials involving ICIs and are often not offered therapy because evidence is lacking in this patient population. More recent data, however, suggest that patients with an autoimmune condition – even those with active disease at the time of ICI initiation – may be safely treated.[5]

Physicians should weigh the benefits and risks when considering treatment with ICIs. If treated, patients should be closely monitored for recurrence or exacerbation of the underlying autoimmune condition;[6] a multidisciplinary approach to care should be adopted that includes other specialists involved in the management of the patient's autoimmune condition.[5]

Key points – optimizing patient care and early recognition of immune-related adverse events

- Engagement with emergency physicians is essential to ensure immune-related toxicity of therapy is considered in patients presenting to hospital.
- A multidisciplinary approach to management of immune-related adverse events is required and, where possible, specialists with an interest in immune checkpoint inhibitor (ICI) toxicities should be identified.
- Comprehensive baseline education should be provided before ICI treatment is started.
- Nurses have a pivotal role in the care and management of patients using ICIs, including education, assessment, monitoring, coordination and support.
- ICIs can be considered in patients with pre-existing autoimmune conditions, but these individuals should be monitored closely and cared for by a multidisciplinary team.

Key references

1. Lomax AJ, McNeil C. Acute management of autoimmune toxicity in cancer patients on immunotherapy: common toxicities and the approach for the emergency physician. *Emerg Med Australas* 2017;29:245–51.

2. Hryniewicki AT, Wang C, Shatsky R, Coyne CJ. Management of immune checkpoint inhibitor toxicities: a review and clinical guideline for emergency physicians. *J Emerg Med* 2018;55:489–502.

3. Davies M, Duffield EA. Safety of checkpoint inhibitors for cancer treatment: strategies for patient monitoring and management of immune-mediated adverse events. *Immunotargets Ther* 2017;6:51–71.

4. Nagai H, Muto M. Optimal management of immune-related adverse events resulting from treatment with immune-checkpoint inhibitors: a review and update. *Int J Clin Onc* 2018;23:410–20.

5. Abdel-Wahab N, Shah M, Lopez-Olivio MA, Suarez-Almazor ME. Use of immune checkpoint inhibitors in the treatment of patients with cancer and preexisting autoimmune disease. *Ann Intern Med* 2018;168:121–30.

6. Brahmer JR, Lacchetti C, Schneider BJ et al. Management of immune-related adverse events in patients treated with immune checkpoint inhibitor therapy: American Society of Clinical Oncology Clinical Practice Guideline. *J Clin Oncol* 2018;36:1714–68.

8 Management summaries

Having discussed the need for vigilance and the management principles for key immune-related adverse events (irAEs) in Chapters 2 to 6, in this chapter we provide summarized guidelines for the management of irAEs, alongside the grading criteria for each irAE.

Notes and abbreviations:

†Instrumental activities of daily living (ADL) are the activities and tasks beyond basic self-care that are necessary for living independently; they include activities such as using the telephone, cleaning the house, doing laundry, shopping, going to the bank and managing medications.

‡Self-care ADL are bathing, dressing and undressing, self-feeding, using the toilet and taking medications; not bedridden.

ADL: activities of daily living

ALT: alanine transaminase

AST: aspartate transaminase

BSA: body surface area

CK: creatine kinase

CT: computed tomography

CTLA-4: cytotoxic T lymphocyte-associated antigen

ECG: electrocardiogram

ft_3: (free) triiodothyronine

fT_4: free thyroxine

GABA: γ-aminobutyric acid;

ICI: immune checkpoint inhibitor

ICU: intensive care unit

IL: interleukin

IVIG: intravenous immunoglobulin

NSAID: non-steroidal anti-inflammatory drug

PD-1: programmed cell death 1 protein

PD-L1: programmed cell death ligand 1

TNF: tumor necrosis factor

TSH: thyroid-stimulating hormone

ULN: upper limit of normal

TABLE 8.1

Management of immune-related colitis*
See Chapter 2, pages 24–8

Grade of colitis	Management
Grade 1	
• Asymptomatic	• Continue ICI
• Clinical or diagnostic observations only	• Educate patient and family about escalating signs and symptoms of colitis
• Intervention not indicated	• Monitor symptoms closely
	• Antidiarrheal medication if required
	• Monitor for dehydration
Grade 2	
• Abdominal pain	• Stop ICI until symptoms reduce to grade 1
• Mucus or blood in stool	• Stool and blood work-up
	• Gastroenterologist consultation
	• Consider hospitalization
	• Prednisone (or methylprednisolone equivalent), 1 mg/kg/day
	• Consider escalation of prednisone to 2 mg/kg/day if no improvement in symptoms
	• Taper steroids slowly over 4–6 weeks
	• Restart ICI on improvement of symptoms to grade 1 and taper steroids to < 10 mg/day
Grade 3	
• Severe abdominal pain	• Permanently discontinue CTLA-4 ICI and stop PD-1/PD-L1 ICI until symptoms reduce to grade 1
• Peritoneal signs	• Stool and blood work-up
	• Gastroenterologist consultation
	• Hospitalization recommended
	• Prednisone (or methylprednisolone equivalent), 1 mg/kg/day, with escalation to 2 mg/kg/day if refractory or no improvement for 3 days
	• Escalate to intravenous infliximab, 5 mg/kg, if refractory to steroids after 3 days

CONTINUED

TABLE 8.1 (CONTINUED)

Management of immune-related colitis*
See Chapter 2, pages 24–8

Grade of colitis	Management
Grade 4 • Life-threatening consequences • Urgent intervention indicated	• Permanently discontinue ICI • Admit to hospital • Stool and blood work-up • Gastroenterologist consultation • Intravenous steroids, 1–2 mg/kg/day, with a slow taper over 4–6 weeks once symptoms reach grade 1 • Intravenous infliximab, 5 mg/kg (dose 1) and 10 mg/kg (dose 2), if refractory to steroids after 3–5 days • Second dose of intravenous infliximab after 2 weeks if needed

Bullets within a grade are the equivalent of 'or'.
*A disorder characterized by inflammation of the colon.
For grading definitions see Table 2.1. For an explanation of abbreviations see page 73.
Adapted from Puzanov et al. 2017 and National Institutes of Health, National Cancer Institute 2017.[1,2]

TABLE 8.2

Management of immune-related hepatitis
See Chapter 2, pages 28–30

Grade of hepatitis	Management
Grade 1 • Asymptomatic • AST, ALT > ULN to ×3 ULN • Total bilirubin > ULN to ×1.5 ULN	• Continue ICI • Monitor liver function once or twice a week
Grade 2 • Asymptomatic • AST, ALT > ×3 to < ×5 ULN • Total bilirubin > ×1.5 to < ×3 ULN	• Stop ICI until liver function variables fall to grade 1 • Undertake work-up to rule out other etiologies • Prednisone, 0.5–1 mg/kg/day (or methylprednisolone equivalent) • Monitor liver function twice a week • Consider liver CT or ultrasound • Taper steroids slowly over 4–6 weeks • Restart ICI on improvement of symptoms to grade 1 and taper steroids to < 10 mg/day
Grade 3 • Symptomatic liver dysfunction • Fibrosis by biopsy • Compensated cirrhosis • Reactivation of chronic hepatitis • AST, ALT ×5 to ×20 ULN • Total bilirubin ×3 to ×10 ULN	• Permanently discontinue ICI • Monitor liver function every 1–2 days • Administer prednisone (or methylprednisolone equivalent), 1–2 mg/kg/day • If refractory or no improvement after 3 days, consider mycophenolate mofetil • Consider liver CT or ultrasound • Consider liver biopsy • Taper steroids slowly over 4–6 weeks

CONTINUED

TABLE 8.2 (CONTINUED)

Management of immune-related hepatitis
See Chapter 2, pages 28–30

Grade of hepatitis	Management
Grade 4	
• Decompensated liver function (e.g. ascites, coagulopathy, encephalopathy, coma) • AST, ALT > ×20 ULN • Total bilirubin > ×10 ULN	• Permanently discontinue ICI • Monitor liver function every 1–2 days • Administer prednisone (or methylprednisolone equivalent), 1–2 mg/kg/day • If refractory or no improvement after 3 days, consider mycophenolate mofetil • Consider liver CT or ultrasound • Consider liver biopsy • Taper steroids slowly over 4–6 weeks

For an explanation of abbreviations see page 73.

Sources: Puzanov et al. 2017 and Brahmer et al. 2018.[1,3]

TABLE 8.3

Management of immune-related maculopapular rash*
See Chapter 3, pages 33–4, 36–9

Grade of rash	Management
Grade 1	
• Macules/papules covering < 10% BSA with or without symptoms (e.g. pruritus, burning, tightness)	• Continue ICI • Educate patient and family about escalating signs and symptoms and self-management strategies • Oral antihistamine (e.g. loratadine,10 mg daily) • Topical corticosteroids
Grade 2	
• Macules/papules covering 10–30% BSA with or without symptoms (e.g. pruritus, burning, tightness) • Limiting instrumental ADL[†] • Rash covering > 30% BSA with or without mild symptoms	• Continue ICI • Educate patient and family about escalating signs and symptoms and self-management strategies • Oral antihistamine (e.g. loratadine, 10 mg daily) • Topical corticosteroids • Non-urgent dermatology referral
Grade 3	
• Macules/papules covering > 30% BSA with moderate or severe symptoms • Limiting self-care ADL[‡]	• Stop ICI • Educate patient and family about escalating signs and symptoms and self-management strategies • Oral antihistamine (e.g. loratadine, 10 mg daily) • Initiate same-day dermatologist consultation • Systemic corticosteroids: prednisone (or methylprednisolone equivalent), 0.5–1 mg/kg/day, until resolution to < grade 1, with slow tapering on resolution

Bullets within a grade are the equivalent of 'or'.
*A disorder characterized by the presence of macules (flat) and papules (elevated).
For ADL[†‡] definitions and an explanation of abbreviations see page 73.
Sources: Puzanov et al. 2017, National Institutes of Health, National Cancer Institute 2017, and Haanen et al. 2017.[1,2,4]

TABLE 8.4

Management of immune-related pruritus*
See Chapter 3, pages 34, 36–9

Grade of pruritus	Management
Grade 1	
• Mild or localized • Topical intervention indicated	• Oral antihistamine (e.g. loratadine, 10 mg daily – non-sedating; hydroxyzine, 10–25 mg four times a day or at bedtime) • Emollients with cream or ointment base • Topical corticosteroid
Grade 2	
• Widespread and intermittent • Skin changes from scratching (e.g. edema, papulation, excoriations, lichenification, oozing/crusts) • Oral intervention indicated • Limiting instrumental ADL[†]	• Oral antihistamine (e.g. loratadine, 10 mg daily – non-sedating; hydroxyzine, 10–25 mg four times a day or at bedtime) • Emollients with cream or ointment base • Topical corticosteroid • Dermatology referral • Oral corticosteroids: prednisone (or methylprednisolone equivalent), 0.5–1 mg/kg/day tapered over 2 weeks
Grade 3	
• Widespread and constant • Limiting self-care ADL[‡] or sleep • Systemic corticosteroid or immunosuppressive therapy indicated	• Dermatology referral • Oral corticosteroids: prednisone (or methylprednisolone equivalent), 0.5–1 mg/kg/day tapered over 2 weeks • GABA agonist (pregabalin, gabapentin, 100–300 mg three times a day)

Bullets within a grade are the equivalent of 'or'.
*A disorder characterized by an intense itching sensation.
For ADL[†‡] definitions and an explanation of abbreviations see page 73.
Sources: Puzanov et al. 2017, National Institutes of Health, National Cancer Institute 2017, and Haanen et al. 2017.[1,2,4]

TABLE 8.5

Management of bullous dermatoses*
See Chapter 3, pages 36–9

Grade of bullous dermatoses	Management
Grade 1 • Asymptomatic • Blisters covering < 10% BSA • No associated erythema	• Continue ICI if blisters < 10% BSA and non-inflammatory • Local wound care where necessary • Educate patient and family about escalating signs and symptoms and self-management strategies
Grade 2 • Blistering that affects quality of life and requires intervention based on diagnosis not meeting criteria for grade > 2 • Blisters covering 10–30% BSA	• Stop ICI • Educate patient and family about escalating signs and symptoms and self-management strategies • Refer to dermatology for work-up and to guide appropriateness of resuming ICI • Wound care • Class 1 high-potency topical corticosteroid (e.g. betamethasone or equivalent) with reassessment every 3 days for signs of progression or improvement • Escalate to systemic corticosteroids if no improvement after 3 days (prednisone, 0.5–1 mg/kg/day, with a slow taper over 4 weeks) • Manage symptoms as necessary (e.g. pain, fever)
Grade 3 • Skin sloughing covering > 30% BSA • Associated pain • Limiting self-care ADL[‡]	• Stop ICI • Refer to dermatology for work-up and to guide appropriateness of resuming ICI • Wound care • Intravenous corticosteroids (methylprednisolone), 1–2 mg/kg/day, tapering over at least 4 weeks • Manage symptoms as necessary (e.g. pain, fever)

CONTINUED

TABLE 8.5 (CONTINUED)

Management of bullous dermatoses*
See Chapter 3, pages 36–9

Grade of bullous dermatoses	Management
Grade 4	
• Blisters covering > 30% BSA • Associated fluid or electrolyte abnormalities	• Permanent discontinuation of ICI • Admit to hospital with urgent dermatology referral to supervise management • Intravenous corticosteroids (methylprednisolone), 1–2 mg/kg/day, tapering over at least 4 weeks • Manage symptoms as necessary (e.g. pain, fever)

*Including bullous pemphigoid or other autoimmune bullous dermatoses.
For ADL[+] definition and an explanation of abbreviations see page 73.
Sources: Puzanov et al. 2017, National Institutes of Health, National Cancer Institute 2017, and Haanen et al. 2017.[1,2,4]

TABLE 8.6

Management of immune-related primary hypothyroidism*
See Chapter 4, pages 43–4, 47–8

Grade	Management
Grade 1 • TSH < 10 mIU/L • Asymptomatic • Clinical or diagnostic observations only • Intervention not indicated	• Continue ICI • Close monitoring of TSH, fT_4
Grade 2 • TSH persistently > 10 mIU/L • Symptomatic • Thyroid replacement indicated • Limiting instrumental ADL[†]	• Consider stopping ICI until symptoms resolve to baseline • Endocrine consultation • Start thyroid hormone replacement in symptomatic patients with any degree of TSH elevation or in asymptomatic patients with persistent TSH levels > 10 mIU/L (measured 4 weeks apart) • Repeat TSH and fT_4 levels every 6–8 weeks • Monitor thyroid function at least every 6 weeks once ICI has been restarted
Grade 3 • Severe symptoms • Limiting self-care ADL[‡] • Hospitalization indicated	• Stop ICI until symptoms resolve • Endocrine consultation • Start thyroid hormone replacement • Consider hospital admission for management and monitoring
Grade 4 • Life-threatening consequences • Urgent intervention indicated	• Stop ICI until symptoms resolve • Endocrine consultation • Start thyroid hormone replacement • Admit to hospital for management and monitoring

Bullets within a grade definition are the equivalent of 'or'.
*Elevated TSH, normal or low fT_4. For ADL[†‡] definitions and an explanation of abbreviations see page 73. Sources: Puzanov et al. 2017, National Institutes of Health, National Cancer Institute 2017, and Brahmer et al. 2018.[1–3]

TABLE 8.7

Management of immune-related primary hyperthyroidism*
See Chapter 4, pages 44–5, 47–8

Grade	Management
Grade 1 • Asymptomatic • Clinical or diagnostic observations only • Intervention not indicated	• Continue ICI • Monitor TSH and fT4 every 2–3 weeks until it is evident if hyperthyroidism will persist or transition to hypothyroidism
Grade 2 • Symptomatic • Thyroid suppression therapy indicated • Limiting instrumental ADL†	• Consider stopping ICI until symptoms return to baseline • Endocrine consultation • Symptomatic relief (β-blocker) • Hydration and supportive care as indicated • Work-up for Graves' disease where hyperthyroidism persists > 6 weeks
Grade 3 • Severe symptoms • Limiting self-care ADL‡ • Hospitalization indicated	• Stop ICI until symptoms resolve • Endocrine consultation • Symptomatic relief (β-blocker) • Consider hospitalization if concerned for thyroid storm or symptoms are severe • Start prednisone, 1–2 mg/kg/day, with a taper over 1–2 weeks
Grade 4 • Life-threatening consequences • Urgent intervention indicated	• Stop ICI until symptoms resolve • Endocrine consultation • Symptomatic relief (β-blocker) • Consider hospitalization if concerned for thyroid storm or symptoms are severe • Start prednisone, 1–2 mg/kg/day, with a taper over 1–2 weeks

*Suppressed TSH and high, normal or elevated fT_4 and/or fT_3. For ADL†‡ definitions and an explanation of abbreviations see page 73. Sources: Puzanov et al. 2017; National Institutes of Health, National Cancer Institute 2017, and Brahmer et al. 2018.[1–3]

TABLE 8.8

Management of immune-related hypophysitis*
See Chapter 4, pages 45–6, 47–8

Grade of hypophysitis	Management
Grade 1	
• Asymptomatic or mild symptoms • Clinical or diagnostic observations only • Intervention not indicated	• Stop ICI • Endocrine consultation • Start replacement hormones with dosing as in hypothyroidism and adrenal insufficiency guidelines • Ensure corticosteroids are started several days before thyroid hormone to prevent adrenal crisis
Grade 2	
• Moderate symptoms • Minimal, local or non-invasive intervention indicated • Limiting instrumental ADL†	• Stop ICI • Endocrine consultation • Start replacement hormones with dosing as in hypothyroidism and adrenal insufficiency guidelines • Ensure corticosteroids are started several days before thyroid hormone to prevent adrenal crisis
Grade 3	
• Severe or medically significant but not immediately life-threatening • Hospitalization indicated • Limiting self-care ADL‡	• Stop ICI • Endocrine consultation • Start replacement hormones with dosing as in hypothyroidism and adrenal insufficiency guidelines • Ensure corticosteroids are started several days before thyroid hormone to prevent adrenal crisis • Consider pulse dose therapy with prednisone, 1–2 mg/kg oral daily (or equivalent), with a taper over at least 2 weeks

CONTINUED

TABLE 8.8 (CONTINUED)

Management of immune-related hypophysitis*
See Chapter 4, pages 45–6, 47–8

Grade of hypophysitis	Management
Grade 4 • Life-threatening consequences • Urgent intervention indicated	• Stop ICI • Endocrine consultation • Start replacement hormones with dosing as in hypothyroidism and adrenal insufficiency guidelines • Ensure corticosteroids are started several days before thyroid hormone to prevent adrenal crisis • Consider pulse dose therapy with prednisone, 1–2 mg/kg oral daily (or equivalent), with a taper over at least 2 weeks

*Inflammation of the pituitary with associated deficiencies in some or all anterior pituitary hormones.

For ADL[†‡] definitions and an explanation of abbreviations see page 73.

Sources: Puzanov et al. 2017, National Institutes of Health, National Cancer Institute 2017, and Brahmer et al. 2018.[1–3]

TABLE 8.9

Management of immune-related primary adrenal insufficiency*
See Chapter 4, pages 46, 47–8

Grade	Management
Grade 1	
• Asymptomatic • Clinical or diagnostic observations only • Intervention not indicated	• Consider stopping ICI until stable on hormone replacement • Endocrine consultation • Prednisone, 5–10 mg daily, or hydrocortisone, 10–20 mg orally morning and 5–10 mg orally early afternoon • Fludrocortisone, 0.1 mg/day, may be indicated for mineralocorticoid replacement • Titrate as indicated
Grade 2	
• Moderate symptoms • Medical intervention indicated	• Consider stopping ICI until stable on hormone replacement • Endocrine consultation • Prednisone, 20 mg daily, or hydrocortisone, 20–30 mg morning and 10–20 mg afternoon
Grade 3	
• Severe symptoms • Hospitalization indicated	• Stop ICI • Admit to hospital for management • Endocrine consultation • Intravenous normal saline (2 L minimum) • Intravenous stress-dose corticosteroids (hydrocortisone, 100 mg, or dexamethasone, 4 mg) • Taper stress-dose corticosteroids down to maintenance doses (as for grade 1)

CONTINUED

TABLE 8.9 (CONTINUED)

Management of immune-related primary adrenal insufficiency*

See Chapter 4, pages 46, 47–8

Grade	Management
Grade 4	
• Life-threatening consequences • Urgent intervention indicated	• Stop ICI • Admit to hospital for management • Endocrine consultation • Intravenous normal saline (2 L minimum) • Intravenous stress-dose corticosteroids (hydrocortisone, 100 mg, or dexamethasone, 4 mg) • Taper stress-dose corticosteroids down to maintenance doses (as for grade 1)

Bullets within a grade definition are the equivalent of 'or'.

*Adrenal gland failure leading to low cortisol, high adrenocorticotropic hormone (both morning) as well as electrolyte imbalances (hyponatremia and hyperkalemia).

For an explanation of abbreviations see page 73.

Sources: Puzanov et al. 2017; National Institutes of Health, National Cancer Institute 2017, and Brahmer et al. 2018.[1–3]

TABLE 8.10

Management of immune-related type 1 diabetes*
See Chapter 4, pages 46–8

Grade of type 1 diabetes	Management
Grade 1	
• Asymptomatic or mild symptoms • Fasting glucose > ULN–160 mg/dL (> ULN–8.9 mmol/L) • No ketosis or evidence of type 1 diabetes	• Continue ICI with close clinical and biochemical follow-up
Grade 2	
• Moderate symptoms • Fasting glucose > 160–250 mg/dL (> 8.9–13.9 mmol/L) • Ketosis or evidence of type 1 diabetes	• Stop ICI until glucose levels are controlled • Start insulin • Urgent endocrine consultation • Admit to hospital in cases of diabetic ketoacidosis
Grade 3	
• Severe symptoms • Medically significant • Fasting glucose > 250–500 mg/dL (> 13.9–27.8 mmol/L)	• Stop ICI until glucose levels are controlled • Urgent endocrine consultation • Start insulin • Admit to hospital for management • Monitor for signs of diabetic ketoacidosis

CONTINUED

TABLE 8.10 (CONTINUED)

Management of immune-related type 1 diabetes*
See Chapter 4, pages 46–8

Grade of type 1 diabetes	Management
Grade 4	
• Severe symptoms • Life-threatening • Fasting glucose > 500 mg/dL (> 27.8 mmol/L)	• Stop ICI until glucose levels are controlled • Urgent endocrine consultation • Start insulin • Hospital admission for management • Monitor for signs of diabetic ketoacidosis

Bullets within a grade definition are the equivalent of 'or'.
*Defined as hyperglycemia in the National Cancer Institute's Common Terminology Criteria for Adverse Events.
For an explanation of abbreviations see page 73.
Sources: Puzanov et al. 2017, National Institutes of Health, National Cancer Institute 2017, and Brahmer et al. 2018.[1–3]

TABLE 8.11

Management of immune-related pneumonitis*
See Chapter 5, pages 51–3, 54–6

Grade of pneumonitis	Management
Grade 1	
• Asymptomatic	• Stop ICI
• Confined to one lobe of the lung or < 25% of lung parenchyma	• Re-image at least prior to every cycle of ICI (at least every 3 weeks)
	– If resolution of pulmonary infiltrates is demonstrated, resume therapy with close follow-up of symptoms
• Clinical or diagnostic observations only	– If evidence of progression, treat as higher grade
	– If no change, consider restarting treatment with close follow-up of new symptoms
	• Monitor patients weekly with history, physical examination and pulse oximetry
Grade 2	
• Symptomatic	• Withhold ICI until resolution to grade 1
• Involves more than one lobe of the lung or 25–50% of lung parenchyma	• Consider admission to hospital
	• Respiratory specialist consultation and consider referral to infectious disease specialist
• Medical intervention indicated	• Prednisone, 1–2 mg/kg/day (or methylprednisolone equivalent), taper by 5–10 mg/week over 4–6 weeks if symptoms have improved after 48–72 hours of corticosteroids/supportive care
• Limiting instrumental ADL[†]	
	• Consider bronchoscopy
	• Consider empirical antibiotics
	• If no clinical improvement after 48–72 hours, treat as grade 3

CONTINUED

TABLE 8.11 (CONTINUED)

Management of immune-related pneumonitis*
See Chapter 5, pages 51–3, 54–6

Grade of pneumonitis	Management
Grade 3	

• Severe symptoms
• Hospitalization required
• Involves all lung lobes or > 50% of lung parenchyma
• Limiting self-care ADL[‡]
• Oxygen indicated
	• Permanently discontinue ICI
	• Admit to hospital and consider ICU care
	• Respiratory and infectious disease specialist consultations
	• Bronchoscopy with bronchoalveolar lavage
	• Empirical antibiotics
	• Intravenous methylprednisolone, 1–2 mg/kg/day
	• If no improvement after 48 hours, add one of:
	  – Infliximab, 5 mg/kg
	  – Intravenous mycophenolate mofetil, 1 g twice a day
	  – Intravenous immunoglobulin for 5 days
	  – Cyclophosphamide
	• Taper steroids over 4–6 weeks

Grade 4	

• Life-threatening respiratory compromise
• Urgent intervention indicated (intubation)
	• Permanently discontinue ICI
	• Admit to hospital and consider ICU care
	• Respiratory and infectious disease specialist consultations
	• Bronchoscopy with bronchoalveolar lavage
	• Empirical antibiotics
	• Intravenous methylprednisolone, 1–2 mg/kg/day
	• If no improvement after 48 hours, add one of:
	  – Infliximab, 5 mg/kg
	  – Intravenous mycophenolate mofetil, 1 g twice a day
	  – Intravenous immunoglobulin for 5 days
	  – Cyclophosphamide
	• Taper steroids over 4–6 weeks

*Focal or diffuse inflammation of the lung parenchyma. For ADL[†‡] definitions and an explanation of abbreviations see page 73.
Sources: Puzanov et al. 2017, and Brahmer et al. 2018.[1,3]

TABLE 8.12

Management of sarcoidosis*

See Chapter 5, pages 53–4

Stage of sarcoidosis	Management
Stage 0 • No adenopathy or infiltrates	• No treatment
Stage 1 • Hilar and mediastinal adenopathy only	• No treatment
Stage 2 • Adenopathy and pulmonary infiltrates	• Stop ICI • Consider treatment with corticosteroids • Consider further immunosuppression
Stage 3 • Pulmonary infiltrates only	• Stop ICI • Consider treatment with corticosteroids • Consider further immunosuppression
Stage 4 • Pulmonary fibrosis	• Stop ICI • Consider treatment with corticosteroids • Consider further immunosuppression

*Grades not defined in the National Cancer Institute's Common Terminology Criteria for Adverse Events (nothing specified). Management is based on standard management guidelines of sarcoidosis in the general population – for example, Baughman et al. 2011.[5]

TABLE 8.13

Management of immune-related nephritis*
See Chapter 6, pages 58–9

Grade of nephritis	Management
Grade 1	
• Creatinine ×1.5–2.0 above baseline	• Stop ICI while other etiologies are excluded
Grade 2	
• Creatinine ×2–3 above baseline	• Stop ICI until resolution to grade 1
	• Nephrology consultation
	• Intravenous hydration
	• Exclude other etiologies and, if no other cause identified, start prednisone, 0.5–1 mg/kg/day, or equivalent
	• If no improvement, or worsening, then increase to prednisone, 1–2 mg/kg/day, or equivalent, and permanently discontinue ICI
	• If improvement to grade 1, taper steroids over 4–6 weeks and consider restarting ICI therapy once steroid dose < 10 mg
Grade 3	
• Creatinine > ×3 above baseline	• Permanently discontinue ICI
• Hospitalization indicated	• Admit to hospital
	• Nephrology consultation
	• Prednisone, 1–2 mg/kg/day, or equivalent
	• Slow taper of steroids over 4–6 weeks
Grade 4	
• Life-threatening consequences	• Permanently discontinue ICI
• Dialysis indicated	• Admit to hospital
	• Nephrology consultation
	• Prednisone, 1–2 mg/kg/day, or equivalent
	• Slow taper of steroids over 4–6 weeks

*Inflammation of the kidney affecting the structure. For an explanation of abbreviations see page 73.
Sources: Puzanov et al. 2017, National Institutes of Health, National Cancer Institute 2017, Brahmer et al. 2018, Haanen et al. 2017.[1-4]

TABLE 8.14

Management of immune-related inflammatory arthritis*
See Chapter 6, pages 59–60

Grade of inflammatory arthritis	Management
Grade 1	
• Mild pain with inflammation, erythema or joint swelling	• Continue ICI • Start analgesics: NSAIDs
Grade 2	
• Moderate pain associated with signs of inflammation, erythema or joint swelling, limiting instrumental ADL[†]	• Stop ICI • Rheumatology consultation • Escalate analgesia • Consider prednisone or prednisolone, 10–20 mg/day, for 4–6 weeks • If no improvement in 4–6 weeks, escalate to grade 3 management, otherwise slowly taper steroids • Consider intra-articular corticosteroid injection for large joints
Grade 3–4	
• Severe pain associated with signs of inflammation, erythema or joint swelling • Irreversible joint damage • Disabling • Limiting self-care ADL[‡]	• Stop ICI and only consider restarting ICI therapy in consultation with a rheumatologist and when symptoms have reached grade 1 • Rheumatology consultation • Initiate oral prednisone, 0.5–1 mg/kg • If no improvement within 4 weeks, consider additional immunosuppressive therapy such as methotrexate (with folic acid supplementation), TNF inhibition or IL-6 receptor antibody (tocilizumab)

*A disorder characterized by inflammation of the joints. For ADL[†‡] definitions and an explanation of abbreviations see page 73.
Sources: Puzanov et al. 2017, National Institutes of Health, National Cancer Institute 2017, Brahmer et al. 2018, Kim et al. 2017.[1–3,6]

TABLE 8.15

Management of immune-related myositis*
See Chapter 6, pages 59–60

Grade of myositis	Management
Grade 1	
• Mild weakness with or without pain	• Continue ICI • If CK is elevated and patient has muscle weakness treat as grade 2 and consider oral steroids • Analgesia as required
Grade 2	
• Moderate weakness with or without pain • Limiting age-appropriate instrumental ADL[†]	• Stop ICI • Rheumatology or neurology consultation • Analgesia with NSAID • If CK is elevated (×3 or more) initiate prednisone, 0.5–1 mg/kg • ICI may be resumed once symptoms are controlled and if CK is normal and prednisone is < 10 mg
Grade 3–4	
• Severe weakness with or without pain • Limiting self-care ADL[‡]	• Stop ICI • Consider admission to hospital • Urgent referral to rheumatology or neurology • Prednisone, 1 mg/kg, or equivalent • Consider methylprednisolone, 1–2 mg/kg, intravenously if severe compromise • Consider plasmapheresis • Consider IVIG therapy • If no improvement of symptoms and/or CK levels after 4–6 weeks, consider other immunosuppressive agents such as methotrexate or mycophenolate mofetil

*A disorder characterized by muscle inflammation with weakness and elevated muscle enzymes (CK). Muscle pain can be present in severe cases and can be life-threatening if respiratory muscles or myocardium are involved.

For ADL[†‡] definitions and an explanation of abbreviations see page 73.

Sources: Puzanov et al. 2017, National Institutes of Health, National Cancer Institute 2017, Brahmer et al. 2018, Kim et al. 2017.[1–3,6]

TABLE 8.16

Management of immune-related polymyalgia-like syndrome*
See Chapter 6, pages 59–60

Grade of polymyalgia-like syndrome	Management
Grade 1	
• Mild stiffness and pain	• Continue ICI
	• Analgesia as required
Grade 2	
• Moderate stiffness and pain, limiting age-appropriate instrumental ADL[†]	• Stop ICI until grade 1 and/or prednisone < 10 mg
	• Prednisone, 20 mg/day, or equivalent, tapering steroids over 3–4 weeks when symptoms improve
	• Rheumatology referral
Grade 3–4	
• Severe stiffness and pain, limiting self-care ADL[‡]	• Stop ICI and consider restarting when symptoms reach grade 1 and in consultation with a rheumatologist
	• Rheumatology referral
	• Prednisone, 20 mg/day, or equivalent
	• Consider steroid-sparing agent such as methotrexate if prolonged steroids are indicated

*Characterized by marked pain and stiffness in proximal upper and/or lower extremities and no signs of true muscle inflammation such as CK elevation or findings of myositis.
For ADL[†‡] definitions and an explanation of abbreviations see page 73.
Sources: Puzanov et al. 2017, National Institutes of Health, National Cancer Institute 2017, Brahmer et al. 2018, Kim et al. 2017. [1–3,6]

TABLE 8.17

Management of immune-related uveitis*
See Chapter 6, pages 61–2

Grade of uveitis	Management
Grade 1	
• Asymptomatic	• Continue ICI
	• Ophthalmologist referral within 1 week
	• Consider artificial tears
Grade 2	
• Medical intervention required, anterior uveitis	• Stop ICI – may restart once symptoms return to grade 1 or systemic steroids < 10 mg
	• Urgent ophthalmologist referral
	• Topical or systemic corticosteroids
Grade 3	
• Posterior or pan-uveitis	• Permanently discontinue ICI
	• Urgent ophthalmologist consultation
	• Systemic corticosteroids
	• Intravitreal/periocular/topical corticosteroids
Grade 4	
• Vision ≤ 20/200	• Permanently discontinue ICI
	• Urgent ophthalmologist consultation
	• Systemic corticosteroids (intravenous prednisone, 1–2 mg/kg, or methylprednisolone, 0.8–1.6 mg/kg)
	• Intravitreal/periocular/topical corticosteroids as per ophthalmologist

*Inflammation of the middle layer of the eye.
Source: Brahmer et al. 2018.[3]

TABLE 8.18

Management of immune-related episcleritis*
See Chapter 6, pages 61–2

Grade criteria	Management
Grade 1	
• Asymptomatic	• Continue ICI
	• Ophthalmologist referral within 1 week
	• Consider artificial tears
Grade 2	
• Vision ≥ 20/40	• Withhold ICI
	• Urgent ophthalmologist referral
	• Topical or systemic corticosteroids
Grade 3	
• Symptomatic	• Permanently discontinue ICI
• Vision < 20/40	• Urgent ophthalmologist consultation
	• Systemic corticosteroids
	• Topical corticosteroids with cycloplegic agents
Grade 4	
• Vision ≤ 20/200	• Permanently discontinue ICI
	• Urgent ophthalmologist consultation
	• Systemic corticosteroids
	• Topical corticosteroids with cycloplegic agents

*Inflammation affecting the episcleral tissue between the conjunctiva and the sclera in the absence of infection.
Source: Brahmer et al. 2018.[3]

TABLE 8.19

Management of immune-related blepharitis*
See Chapter 6, pages 61–2

Grade of blepharitis	Management
All grades • There is no formal grading system	• Apply warm compresses • Use lubrication drops • Continue ICI unless symptoms persist

*Inflammation of the eyelid that affects the eyelashes or tear production.
Source: Brahmer et al. 2018.[3]

TABLE 8.20

Management of myocarditis, pericarditis, arrhythmias
See Chapter 6, pages 62–3

Grade	Management
Grade 1 • Abnormal ECG, abnormal cardiac biomarker testing	• Stop ICI in all cases and permanently discontinue in all cases ≥ grade 2
Grade 2 • Abnormal screening tests with mild symptoms	• Cardiology consultation • Admit to hospital • Manage symptoms according to cardiology guidelines
Grade 3 • Moderately abnormal testing, with mild symptoms	• Admit to coronary care unit if troponin elevated • Systemic corticosteroids
Grade 4 • Moderate to severe decompensation, life-threatening conditions	• Additional immunosuppression

For an explanation of abbreviations see page 73.

References

1. Puzanov I, Diab A, Abdallah K et al. Managing toxicities associated with immune checkpoint inhibitors: consensus recommendations from the Society for Immunotherapy of Cancer (SITC) Toxicity Management Working Group. *J Immunother Cancer* 2017;5:95.

2. National Institutes of Health, National Cancer Institute. Common Terminology Criteria for Adverse Events (CTCAE) v.5, November 2017. https://ctep.cancer.gov/protocoldevelopment/electronic_applications/docs/CTCAE_v5_Quick_Reference_8.5x11.pdf, last accessed 2 April 2019.

3. Brahmer JR, Lacchetti C, Schneider BJ et al. Management of immune-related adverse events in patients treated with immune checkpoint inhibitor therapy: American Society of Clinical Oncology Clinical Practice Guideline. *J Clin Oncol* 2018;36:1714–68.

4. Haanen JBAG, Carbonnel F, Robert C et al. Management of toxicities from immunotherapy: ESMO Clinical Practice Guidelines for diagnosis, treatment and follow-up. *Ann Oncol* 2017;28(suppl 4):iv119–42.

5. Baughman RP, Culver DA, Judson MA. A concise review of pulmonary sarcoidosis. *Am J Respir Crit Care Med* 2011;183:573–81.

6. Kim ST, Tayar J, Trinh VA et al. Successful treatment of arthritis induced by checkpoint inhibitors with tocilizumab: a case series. *Ann Rheum Dis* 2017;76:2061–4.

Useful resources

American Society of Clinical Oncology
Patient info: +1 571 483 1780
contactus@cancer.net
www.cancer.net

Clinical Oncology Society of Australia
Tel: +61 (02) 8063 4100
cosa@cancer.org.au
www.cosa.org.au

Conquer Cancer Foundation
Tel: +1 571 483 1700
info@conquer.org
www.conquercancerfoundation.org
www.asco.org

European Society for Medical Oncology
Tel: +41 (0)91 973 19 00
esmo@esmo.org
www.esmo.org

Multinational Association of Supportive Care in Cancer
mascc.office@mascc.org
www.mascc.org

National Cancer Institute (USA)
Helpline: +1 800 422 6237
www.cancer.gov

National Comprehensive Cancer Network (USA)
Tel: +1 215 690 0300
Patient info: www.nccn.org/patients/default.aspx
www.nccn.org

Guidelines
Brahmer JR, Lacchetti C, Schneider BJ et al. Management of immune-related adverse events in patients treated with immune checkpoint inhibitor therapy: American Society of Clinical Oncology Clinical Practice Guideline. *J Clin Oncol* 2018;36:1714–68.

Haanen JBAG, Carbonnel F, Robert C et al. Management of toxicities from immunotherapy: ESMO Clinical Practice Guidelines for diagnosis, treatment and follow-up. *Ann Oncol* 2017;28(suppl 4):iv119–42.

Thompson JA. New NCCN Guidelines: recognition and management of immunotherapy-related toxicity. *J Natl Compr Canc Netw* 2018;16:594–6.

Index